What Everyone should know about Medicines

Second Edition

What Everyone should know about Medicines

Second Edition

Professor Guru Prasad Mohanta
M. Pharm., Ph.D., FIC.
Department of Pharmacy,
Annamalai University, Annamalai Nagar - 608 002
Tamil Nadu

PharmaMed Press
An imprint of Pharma Book Syndicate
A Unit of BSP Books Pvt. Ltd.
4-4-309/316, Giriraj Lane,
Sultan Bazar, Hyderabad - 500 095.

What Everyone should know about Medicines, ***Second Edition***
by Professor Guru Prasad Mohanta

Disclaimer: The author and publisher have taken all reasonable precaution to provide reliable information to the readers. The readers must take appropriate consultation with their doctors for treating any illness or health condition or using any medicine. Neither the author nor the publisher would be held responsible for any damages or harms from using this book. The book is not a substitute of consultation with doctor. The brands of any medicine mentioned in the book are just for illustration purpose only. The author and the publisher do not endorse them.

Published by

Pharma Med PRESS
An Imprint of
Pharma Book Syndicate

PharmaMed Press

An imprint of Pharma Book Syndicate

A Unit of BSP Books Pvt. Ltd.
4-4-309/316, Giriraj Lane, Sultan Bazar, Hyderabad - 500 095.
Phone: 040-23445688, 23445600; Fax: 91+40-23445611
E-mail: info@pharmamedpress.com
www.pharmamedpress.com/pharmamedpress.net

ISBN: 978-93-88305-65-5 (HB)

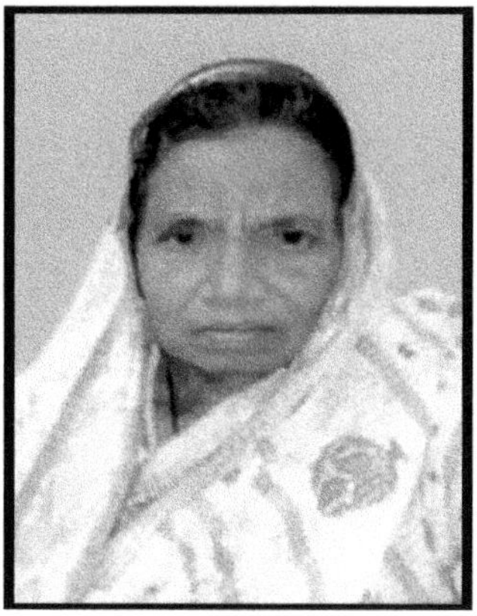

Dedicated to

My mother,

Srimati Sabitri Mohanta

who selflessly worked together with father Late Chakradhar Mohanta to bring us all three brothers to what we are today sacrificing her many personal ambitions and happiness. She was ahead of her times in thought and action. She is a role model of humanity for serving the distressed persons.

Preface to Second Edition

"Education is the most powerful weapon which you can use to change the world."

- Nelson Mandela

With information explosion and improved access to internet, the people are exposed to unlimited source of information. It is really difficult to know which information are accurate, updated and reliable. The consumers often get lost with misleading and unreliable information. This is perhaps a real challenge in medicine related information. One should be careful while browsing through the website and look only the reliable ones. In order to assist the consumers who are interested to know safe and effective use of medicines, I present this second edition of my "What Everyone should know about Medicines". The information is key to successful use of medicines and deriving maximum benefit from medicine use. The word of mouth "More you know about medicines, better do they work for you".

"Don't under estimate the power of a common man". This is not just the popular film dialogue but a movement. The day common people of the country are empowered through education, many of the social ills we face now will be eliminated. The medicines are no exceptions. The real consumers do have very little understanding about the medicines and those who have the knowledge have little time to spare educating the patients on safe and effective use. In this text, I have made attempts to empower the common men with basic knowledge of using medicines so that they can take informed decision about the use of medicines. The materials presented in the book are not mere writings but are tools to empower the patients.

As assured in the first edition, I have made an attempt to update and revise the text. Many new items are introduced. One of the notable features of the new edition is addition of cartoons in some of the themes. These cartoons are drawn by my student, Mr. Joseph Prince. I appreciate his gesture of drawing these cartoons. Hope the readers would like this value addition.

I appreciate the love and patience of my family: Wife Reena, Son Anupam and Daughter Amrita. Without their cooperation, it would have perhaps not been possible to bring this updated second edition. Mr. Anil Shah of PharmaMed Press deserves special appreciation for encouraging to come with revised edition.

The readers' feedback is most important and I would personally be grateful to them for their patronage and suggestion for improvement. Hope my modest attempt of educating the medicines' users would have some impact in the society.

Guru Prasad Mohanta

E-mail: gpmohanta@hotmail.com

Contents

PART B
Medicine Administration

PART C
Individual Medicines

Part A
General Topics

CHAPTER 1

You as Consumer of Medicine Use (Consumers' Rights)

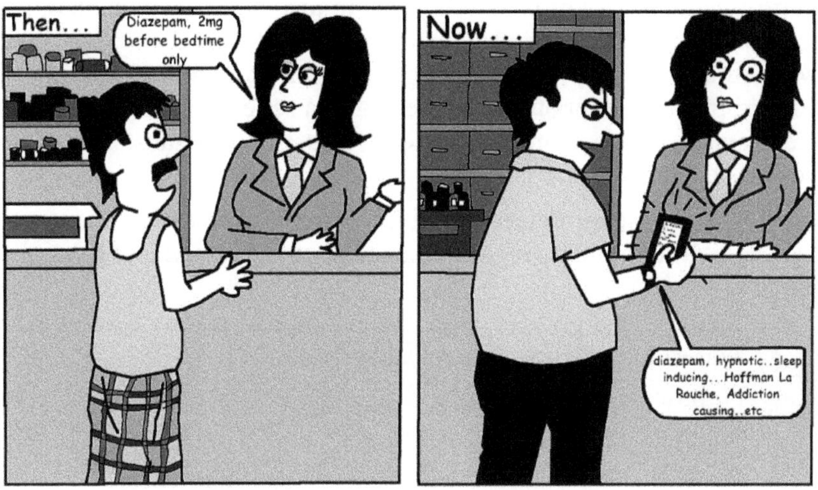
Then...
Diazepam, 2mg before bedtime only
Now...
diazepam, hypnotic..sleep inducing...Hoffman La Rouche. Addiction causing..etc

"Common man must be equipped with knowledge and awareness"

While sitting in a relative's medical store in a small town of Orissa in a hot summer day I found a customer asking, "Why do you give this medicine? It is written not for children". The shopkeeper defenselessly replied it is what your doctor prescribed. This is not an isolated incident.

Gone are the days when only doctors and pharmacists (modern day's compounders) had the privilege of knowing about medicines and the patients were kept dark. The medicine name was used to be written only in Latin. Change in societal perception and patients' attitude towards their well being forced the situation to make patients as a part of their health decision. The consumers (patients) are becoming more active in the treatment of illness, rather than being the passive recipient of therapy. Medicines are probably the most important component of present day treatment. These medicines are double-edged weapons. They are not only very effective but could be dangerous, even fatal, if not used appropriately.

Ask your doctor or pharmacist to know your medicines. It is your right.

Access to information is essential for the consumers to play an active role in drug therapy decision. Informed patients respond more effectively to treatment because of their adherence to medicine use guidelines. Even the consumers can have choice for other brands/medicines (of course with similar activity) based on pricing. In an effort to educate the consumers on appropriate use of medicines a series of educational articles are planned. But a word of caution "This is not a substitute of your doctor's advice".

In order to use medicines effectively, wisely, and safely a consumer is in need of at least following information about the medicines he or she is going to use.

- Name of medicine – generic and brand.
- Purpose of medicine.
- Strength and dose.
- Possible side effects and what should I do if they occur?
- What medicines should not be taken along with this?
- How long to be taken?
- When should be taken?
- What to do if a dose is missed?
- Whether to avoid certain foods or drinks while taking this medicine?
- Whether there is a need to replace any medicine currently taking?
- How to store?

The consumers can get above information either from their doctors or pharmacists. This is their right.

CHAPTER 2

You must know about your Medicine

The medicines are double edged weapons we have to fight against diseases and illness. But they need to be safely used failing which they may even harm us. More we know them better do they work. The medicines are divided into two types: prescription medicines and non-prescription medicines. Irrespective of the types of medicines, one needs to know about the medicines to derive maximum benefit from them and reducing (if not eliminating completely) the harmful effects. No medicine is completely safe for all persons at all times. It is necessary to use them safely and effectively in the best interest of us.

Many of you may have concern about the usefulness of the medicines prescribed to you, the best way to use it, possible side effects, and precautions to observe to avoid complications. Some medicines are required to be taken only after meals, some require to be taken before; some medicines may cause drowsiness disturbing your daily work; your drinking (alcohol) or smoking may interfere with functioning of your medicine. Some of the side effects may not be serious but there may be situation, you need to consult your doctor or need immediate medical attention. Even sometimes you may see duplication of medicines in your prescription.

To use medicines safely, effectively and wisely, one needs to know about the medicines he/she is going to use.

Unfortunately, the information you receive either from your doctor or pharmacist is often far from satisfactory. Just do not go away with the notion: A pill for every ill. Do not follow the advertisements as they are very often misleading and deceptive in nature. There are issues too. You may find it difficult to buy all medicines advised or prescribed, you end up with buying partially. These are not isolated incidents. They have been occurring now and then everywhere. The medicines may not do good but must not harm.

Make sure that you or your family member understands the following before leaving doctor or pharmacy:

- Name of the medicine(s) and the purpose of using them.
- How and when to take your medicine.
- What to do when you miss a dose.
- How long to take the medicine(s).
- Whether your diet or other social habits like drinking or smoking can be continued.
- What are the side effects and what to do if they occur.
- Any special storage requirement at home.

Besides the above information you do need, here are the general safety rules:

- Before starting medications try to find out the causes of your illness.
- Do not follow advertisement.
- Tell your doctor all the medicines you are currently taking.
- Do not stop taking medicines without doctor's advice even if you started feeling better.
- Store your medicines preferably in cool dry place and away from light. Keep away from reach of children.
- If you experience a new symptom after beginning your medicine(s), this may be due to the medicine(s) you are taking or using. Report this to your doctor.
- Discard your old medicines. Never use an expired medicine.
- Do not self medicate unless you are sure of the illness and its remedy.

CHAPTER 3

Names of Medicines

(Medicine -What is in a Name?)

"What is in a Name?" It reminds the Shakespeare's famous drama where Juliet asks "What's in a name? That which we call a rose, by any other name would smell as sweet". She asserted "It is not the name which gives a thing its essential qualities. A name is arbitrary and changing the name does not change Romeo's identity". Perhaps this was true for Juliet and Romeo and their love. But this is not true for your medicine. There is a lot with the name of the medicines!

Look at the name of these medicines: you are prescribed LONA (low sodium salt of Dabur Pharma) for your high blood pressure. But there is one more medicine by the same name LONA (clonazepam of calyx division of Triton Healthcare Private limited). What would your pharmacist do? Will not he get confused? And then guess! Another example: A-Z (multivitamin of Alkem lab) and AZ (azithromycin of Kopran Lab) and ABZ (albendazole of Kare Health Specialities). This is a genuine confusion at pharmacy. But this get further multiplied when doctors' prescription are not legible. The poor patients' fate! The wrong guess could be disastrous. There are many such examples with sound alike and look alike medicines. With multi-ingredient medicines, the problem gets compounded further.

Generic name is universally acceptable. Prescribing in generic name avoids confusion and medication error.

There are three names for each medicine: Chemical name, Generic name and Brand name. All medicines are chemicals. In order to identify them based on their chemical groups, chemical names are given. Chemists or scientists are interested in chemical name. Generic name is also called International Non-Proprietary Name (INN). The generic name is designed by the World Health Organization through defined a procedure. No two medicines have same the same generic name. Generic name is also called common name. Brand name is the trade mark of the individual company. The company spends good amount of resources to promote their brands.

The chemical name and the generic name are same throughout the world. But the brand is different in different countries. The specific brand may not be available in some geographical areas. If the trade mark holder does not market in any country, the same brand is not available there. But the medicine is available in generic name. In USA, there is only one brand for each medicine. Other medicines with same ingredient are available as generics. The generics come to the market after the expiry of the patent period. The generics have to prove experimentally that they have almost the similar effectiveness as the brands before being approved for marketing. In other words, they have been proved to be equal for use as substitution. They are therapeutically equivalent. In India we do not have true brands. What we have are generics, branded generics and brands (for drugs still under patent protection). Lets see an example. Paracetamol is the generic name. There are several branded generics like Crocin, Metacin, Dolo and so on. The company often continues with brand extension: Disprin Plus and Aspro Plus. Disprin and Aspro were known aspirin brands. While the companies stopped marketing aspirin, they extended the same name for paracetamol products. The plus normally signs of something extra but is deceiving altogether with a new substance leave about extra.

As the drugs available in the market are tested and marketed only after compliance report of standard, all drugs available in the market are of good quality. The only difference between the brand and the generic medicine is price. Besides due to confusing and similar names; they are the causes of medication error. On the other hand there are several reports of not of standard quality medicines even in reputed brands.

The time has come for the government to act and define the procedure for granting trade (brand) name in the best interest of patient safety. The well placed guideline and continuing their documentation would help to bring uniformity, clarity and promoting safety of medicines in our country. Branding should not come as misbranding!

CHAPTER 4

Types of Medicines (Dosage Forms)

The active material in a medicine is usually a basic chemical but is as such not given to the patient. This is similar to vegetables that we rarely take raw, but are cooked for food. The active materials are suitably modified or processed to make them suitable for use. This process of conversion requires many other ingredients which are harmless but useful. This is medically called formulation. The active material is formulated into medicines which are available as tablets, capsules, injections etc.

In the formulated form the active material (often called drug) is safe, effective and stable. It helps all the key players of medicine: manufacturers, chemists, prescribers and the patients. Manufacturers can utilize the modern technology to make different forms of medicines and provides opportunities to physicians to prescribe different forms to different patients based on individual need; chemists find them convenient to store for long period and supply them to patients; patients find them convenient for use. The medicine like chloroquine (anti-malarial) is bitter in taste, but is made as syrup for use by children. Insulin, an anti-diabetic, cannot be given by tablets or capsules as it gets destroyed in the stomach and intestine; but is given as injection. Some medicines are formulated to produce only local effects on the skin (ointments), eyes (eye drops), nose (nasal drops) etc. These are few examples of the necessity of formulations.

Oral Dosage Forms: They are meant to be taken through mouth. The administration of medicines through mouth is the simplest, convenient and safest method of using medicines. However, these products are not suitable for patients who have difficulty in swallowing or unconscious or suffering from vomiting. The medicines for children are suitably sweetened and flavoured to make them tastier.

***Capsules*:** The medicinal active ingredients are kept enclosed in shells made of gelatine. Like tablet, each capsule is meant for one dose. There are two types of capsules: hard gelatine capsule and soft gelatine capsule. The hard gelatine capsules generally contain solid materials while soft capsules have solutions, dispersions or liquids of non-aqueous in nature.

Capsules have advantage that the taste of the medicaments are masked and are quicker acting than tablets. They need to be swallowed with glass of water.

Tablets: Each tablet has one dose of the drug. Usually they should be swallowed without breaking with a glass of water.

- Chewable tablets (like Antacids) are to be chewed before swallowing.
- Effervescent tablets (like some Aspirin) are to be added to a glass of water and be drunk while effervescing.
- Sublingual tablets (like isosorbide) are to be kept under tongue. This provides quick relief.

The tablets are also available for use in vagina.

Powders: The medicines in this form are usually not very potent and dose is measured using a spoon. Electrolyte Powders (ORS) are to be dissolved in recommended volume of drinking water. The solution is to be drunk.

Syrups: They are sweetened liquid preparations of unpleasant tasting drugs. The dose should be measured using the supplied spoon only. The sizes of the domestic spoons vary widely. They should be avoided failing which there would be inaccuracy in dosing.

Emulsions: They are liquid preparations of liquid active ingredients. They must be shaken well before measuring a dose. This is written on the label of the product.

Suspensions: They are liquid preparations in which active drugs are not soluble but dispersed in the liquid. They must be shaken well before measuring a dose. This is written on the label of the product.

Dry Syrups (Dry Powders for Syrups): The powders containing the active drugs are supplied in a glass bottle with an instruction to add sufficient drinking water to make syrup. Boiled and cooled water is preferable. You must look for the instruction for making syrups given on the label and do not use after seven days or so as given on the label. Measure dose using the spoon supplied. These drugs are not stable in liquid form and hence supplied as dry powders.

Lozenges: They are large tablets which are not to be swallowed intact. As they dissolve slowly in the mouth, the saliva is to be swallowed slowly. They provide local soothing effect in the mouth or on the irritating throat.

***Mouth Washes*:** They are liquid preparations used in the prevention and treatment of throat infections. When available as concentrated solutions, they should be suitably diluted as given on the label or advised before use. They are not meant for swallowing. Care should be taken not to swallow them in large quantities. They are to be spitted out after use.

Gargles: They are similar to mouth washes but intended for oral hygiene and treat infection of the mouth. Care needs to be taken to avoid swallowing large quantities. They are to be spitted out after use.

Mouth Sprays: These sprays are meant for application to the throat or mouth to relieve conditions like halitosis (bad mouth odour), sore throat, and laryngitis. They are suitably flavoured and contain medicaments such as antiseptics, deodorants etc.

Rectal/Vaginal Dosage Forms: The medicines can be administered to the rectum or vagina for local as well as systemic effects. When it is not practicable for giving medicines by oral administration, they serve as alternative. They require privacy for using these medicines. They must not be swallowed.

Suppositories: They are solid forms often tapered in one end and inserted into rectum. On insertion, they melt or dissolve to give effects.

Pessaries: They are solid forms intended for insertion into vagina where they melt or dissolve to give effects. *Vaginal tablets and capsules are also available for use.*

Inhalation Dosage Forms: They are solutions or suspensions administered by the nasal oral respiratory route for local or systemic effect. Usually they are available as aerosols or metered dose inhalers. They provide quick relief.

***Aerosols (metered dose inhalers)*:** They are pressurized package system containing the medicinally active substance. When activated it releases one dose which is required to be inhaled. One needs to learn the proper technique of using failing which much of the medicines would be lost. They are very quick acting.

Powder for inhalation (Rotacap): The medicinally active substance in powder form is enclosed in a hard capsule. The capsule is to be kept in device called rotahaler. The capsule gets broken during use and the powder is to be inhaled. Mostly used in asthma or chronic obstructive pulmonary airways.

Injection Dosage Forms: They are available as solutions, dispersions or dry powders for making solution or dispersion. They are available as ampoules, vials or plastic pouches or large bottles. Dry powders are mixed with sterile water for injection before administration. They are quick acting compared to oral dosage forms and depending on the types of injection dosage forms they are administered either to a vein, artery, muscle, subcutaneous tissue, eye etc. They are sterile (free from microbes) and patients need the service of a trained person for taking these injections. In case of insulin injections, the patients are trained to take their own injection.

Topically used Dosage Forms: They are administered or applied to the skin. Most of these products are intended for providing local effects on the applied surface (skin). These medicines do belong to antiseptics, antifungal, anti-inflammatory, local anaesthetics, skin emollients and protectants against the effects of sun, wind, pests, and chemical irritants.

Lotions: They are liquid preparations need to be applied on the skin surface. If they are suspensions or emulsions, they require to be shaken well before use. This is written on the label of the product. These preparations are meant for external use only. They are either dabbed on the skin or applied on a suitable dressing and covered with a waterproof dressing to reduce evaporation.

Liniments: They are also liquid preparations like lotions and meant for external application over the skin surface. But they are applied by rubbing on the skin for treating pain and stiffness for underlying musculature. They should not be applied over broken skin, it could be terribly irritating.

Ointments: They are semi-solid preparations intended for external application over the skin. Ointments for application to rectum and nasal mucosa are also available.

Pastes: They are semi-solid preparations like ointments and creams. But these preparations have large proportion of finely powdered solid medicaments and have stiff consistency.

Creams: They are similar to ointments in use but are less greasy and easier to use. They are cosmetically more acceptable than ointments.

Sprays: The topical sprays are intended for application to the skin surface. They are preferred over other topical products because they can be applied without touching. They have medications like for pain relieving, local anaesthetics for sunburn or heat burn, antiseptics, skin protectants and anti-pruritics.

Transdermal patches: They are advanced dosage forms. Though patched over the skin, they are intended for systemic effects. The active medicinal ingredient is slowly released and enters into blood through skin. They are available for treatment of angina, motion sickness, high blood pressure. They are applied at specific site which is mentioned on the label. They provide better patients' compliance than oral medications. The nitroglycerine patch is applied to the arm or chest in the hair free shaven area, scopolamine patch (motion sickness) in behind the ear. They are to be applied several hours before need as it requires sometime to be effective.

Eye, Ear and Nasal Dosage Forms: These preparations are applied topically to the eye, ear and mucous membrane of the nose. These preparations are generally meant for providing local effects. In some instances, the preparations (often with special design) are meant for systemic action. The eye and nasal preparations are used for variety of purpose but the ear products are meant for simply to soften ear wax, to relieve an earache, or to combat ear infection,

Eye Drops: They are sterile preparations meant for instillation into the conjunctival sac. They are available for multi-dose application. Care is necessary not to touch the tip of the container to keep it sterile. Usually one drop is applied at one time and if more than one drop advised wait for one or two minutes before applying the next drop.

Eye Ointments: They are sterile semi-solid preparations meant for application to the conjunctiva or eye lid margin. Care is necessary not to touch the tip of the container to keep it sterile.

Applicaps: They are soft gelatine capsules containing ointments for application to the eye. They are for single use only. The tip of the capsule is to be cut with a clean blade or scissor and the ointment is to be applied.

Ear Drops: They are liquid preparations, usually slightly viscous, meant for instillation into the ear with a dropper. They are used for softening ear wax, relieving an earache or combating ear infection.

Nasal Drops: They are liquids instilled into the nose through use of dropper or through squeezing the plastic bottle. Mostly they are meant for relieving nasal congestion. Long use of these decongestants may cause rebound congestion.

Nasal Sprays: They are used intranasally to relive nasal congestion, inflammation, combat infection and many other purposes. They are quick acting compared to drops.

CHAPTER 5

Branded Vs Generic Medicines

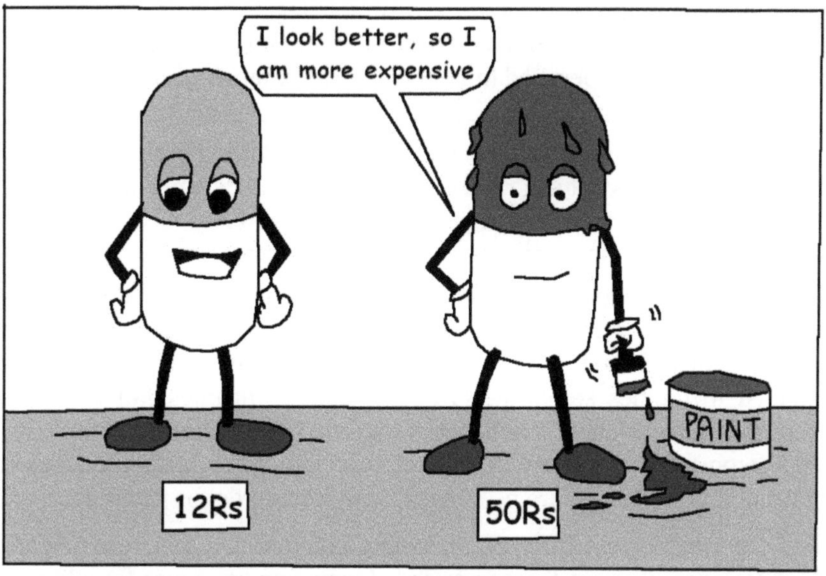
I look better, so I am more expensive
PAINT
12Rs
50Rs

"The only difference between branded and generic is the price"

(a) Branded vs Generic Medicines

When a new medicine (pharmaceutical) is developed and approved for use, the developer pharmaceutical company obtains a patent for exclusive rights for marketing. The company fixes a price and sales the medicine under a trade name called brand name. At present this patent period is 20 years. On expiry of patent period, other companies are at liberty to manufacture the same medicine. They may sell the same under a different brand name of their choice or in common name, known as generic name.

These off patented medicines are called Generic Medicines. The generic medicines are of two types: branded generics and generics.

The quality in terms of purity, effectiveness and safety of branded generics including generics and branded medicines are same. In country like USA, it is essential first to prove that generic medicines are equal in all respects to the innovator's branded product then only they are approved for marketing. The generic manufacturing company establishes this equivalency before applying for product approval for marketing. In our country, though we do not have similar legislative requirement, it is presumed that once medicines are approved for sale they satisfy the minimum standard specified to be maintained in terms of quality.

In absence of adverse reports, the health professionals and the medicine users should realize that the only difference between brand and generic medicine is price.

The pharmaceutical companies want the consumers and doctors to believe that the generics are less of a medicine – less good and less effective than brand named medicines. Study has shown that even branded medicines sometimes from reputed companies fail to comply with all requirements of standards of quality. In absence of a comparative study report, it is important to believe that both branded and generics are of equal quality. There are no lesser quality standards for generics.

Then what is the difference between branded and generics? Usually, the difference between them is price – consumers pay more for a branded product. The companies always set the maximum price possible and spend a lot of money on advertisement convincing health professionals and consumers that their high priced brand named medicines are best. The price differential varies considerably from market to market. In developing countries like India, generic medicines' price is often 50% or less of leading brand, while the price of generics in well developed European market are typically 60-70 % of brand prices. Generic medicine manufacturing stimulates competition reducing the prices.

When brand medicines and their generics are of equal quality, why should a consumer buy brand named medicines paying more. The consumers need to ask the doctor to write generic name of medicines in the prescription. If doctors and pharmacist say the generics are not good, ask why? Is there a guarantee that brand named medicine is of better quality? They may not have interest on generics, as pharma sales persons have frequently impressed them.

In public healthcare delivery systems like government hospitals, the generic medicines only are procured. The drugs and cosmetics act, which regulates the medicine use in our country, stipulates that medicines like ferrous sulphate (a medicine for anemia), analgin, and aspirin etc., should be marketed only on generics.

In absence of adverse reports, the health professionals and consumers should realize that the only difference between a generic and branded medicine is price. Ask for generics and save money.

(b) Generic Prescribing-Whose Dilemma!

In a workshop on promoting generic medicines a senior doctor expressed his views “When we have several brands and generic medicines in the market, they are meant for use. When they are of different price, definitely they do differ in their performance”. Even arguably he continued with an analogy: branded shirts as branded medicines and other shirts with the generic medicines. Branded shirts remain look good after several washings but the other shirts loose the shine just after one or two washes. But what he failed to realize is the medicines and other commodities are not same.

Medicines are different from others. The medicines are regulated commodities. The standards are specified in Drugs and Cosmetics Act and Pharmacopoeias. Every batch of medicines manufactured is tested for quality standard by the manufacturer before being released for distribution (sale). In absence of adverse report, all medicines are of same quality as they comply with the quality standard specified. At the same time there are reports of medicines not of standard quality. This is true for both brands as well generics. One can see the drug controller’s website (cdsco.nic.in) for such reports.

It is not possible for any one including doctors, who prescribe, or chemists, who sell, to identify the defects in quality of medicines without quality checking. A medicine cannot be judged just from its label or packing. In absence of quality defects checked through chemical testing, all medicines available in the market are assumed to be of good quality irrespective of brands or generics. In such situation, how does the doctor infer which product is good and which is not! This is just on basis of individual bias or the briefing of the detailed person (sales executive) of the company.

The price of medicinesin the market varies widely. There are reports of variation as high as 1000%. The price of medicines is one of the contributing factors for our poverty. 39 millions of the country people are pushed to below poverty line every year due to ill health. The average person spends 75% of the health expenditure on medicines. Only one-third of our population has access to essential medicines against the world average of two-third population’s access. Throughout the world, the use of generic medicines is advocated to improve the access especially in resource constrained situations. The resources are always limited.

While the generic prescribing is a solution to the issue of medicines' price and tool to help improving medicines' availability with our limited budget in public hospitals, this is of little value in private practice. If the medicines are prescribed in generics, the chemist would give perhaps the medicines which would give the maximum profit. The consumers have no knowledge of prices of medicines.

The doctors in our society are treated at high esteem. Their role in treatment, saving lives and promoting our health is unquestionable. Often they are considered as God. When the society has such a high faith will they raise to the occasion to help the society further. Here are few issues and facts the doctors should ponder before prescribing a particular brand or product. Brands (available are really branded generics) are costlier than generics. This is because the companies have spent quite large amount in brand promotion and marketing. While we have every respect for the prerogative of the doctors on prescribing, the society does expect a rational behavior from them. The doctor's patient deserves the best. If a doctor believes all brands (products) are not equal, it is understandable that he/she prescribes the trusted brand. But often we see the different brands (of same molecule) are prescribed to different persons by the same doctor. This implies that the individual doctor at least believes some brands (though have no logic) are trust worthy. In such case, will the doctor look at the prices of these brands and prescribe the lowest priced trusted brand to every patient?

It is not just the activists and Governments encourage or direct prescribing in generics. Even the Medical Council of India says "Every physician should, as far as possible, prescribe drugs with generic names and he/she shall ensure that there is a rational prescription and use of drugs". Prescribing in generic names not only improves the medicines access, it also promotes patients safety. The ineligible writing of sound alike and look alike brands leads confusion during dispensing leading to medication errors. The writing the names in generic has many merits.

The medicines are really different from other usable commodities. They do deserve different treatments. The reality is "The one who pays does not decide and one decides does not pay. The one decides is often paid."

CHAPTER 6

Buying Medicines

The modern medicines are not only very effective treating illness, but are toxic and costly too. They are sold in licensed retail units known by various names like: drug store, pharmacy, chemists and druggists. They are sold under the supervision of a pharmacist. It is unsafe to buy medicine from open market, buses, trains or streets corners. It may be fake, adulterated may have expired.

There are two categories of medicines: prescription medicines and over the counter medicines (OTC). The prescription medicines are to be sold only on prescription of doctors, while OTC can be sold without a prescription. Household medicines like simple painkillers, antacids, and fever reducing medicines; come under the category of OTC. The prescription medicines are to be used only under medical advice. However, one can buy any medicine in our country and no prescription is required. It is because of poor drug control measures.

Buy from trusted medical store.
Ask for receipt every time.

The price of medicines varies widely from brand to brand. The consumers need to have price information in hand for selecting a brand or generic. The pharmacist can help them selecting a cheaper alternative (without compromising quality). As per the rule the maximum retail price is written on the label of every pack of medicine. The retailer is not expected to charge more than this price.

It is essential that the consumers buy medicines of appropriate quality at competitive price. Though quality often difficult to check, it is better that the consumers do their part by checking for signs of tempering while buying or using medicines.

The medicines have limited life span and they should not be used once this period is over. They may not be effective or safe to use. The period up to which a medicine can be used is printed on the label as expiry date.

Aggressive and eye catching advertisement, sometimes makes one to buy their medicines trough unreliable and misleading claims. The consumers need to be alert, educative so that they will not fall prey to such unethical advertisements. They should discuss the medicines they wish to buy with the health professionals like doctors and pharmacists. One needs to understand "no medicine is absolutely safe and an element of risk is always involved irrespective of system of medicine".

The following steps by the consumer help him or her best buying:

- Check the name of the medicine(s) – Is it you intend to buy?
- Quality checks: Look very carefully at the outer packing of medicine and also the inner packing as soon as possible after buying.
- Do not buy medicines that show even slightest signs of tempering or do not seem quite right.
- Check the price: The buyers should not pay more than the maximum retail price printed on the package. Some retailers may provide discount because of competition and the buyer needs to take advantage of this.
- Insist on getting a purchase bill or cash memo as a proof of your purchase. This may be required later if a legal action is required to be initiated for claiming compensation for damage caused by the use of medicine.
- Ask the pharmacist: How to use the medicine that one buys?
- Check the expiry date of the product. Do not buy the medicine that is expired or close to the date of expiry.

CHAPTER 7

Medicines' Price

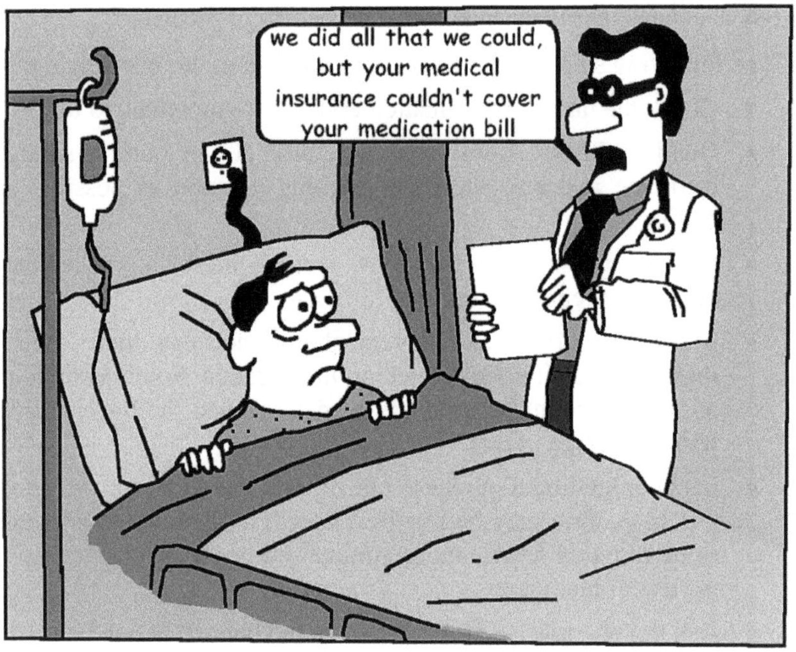
we did all that we could, but your medical insurance couldn't cover your medication bill

It has been reported by the media that the prices of the commonly used medicines like ampicillin (antibiotic), paracetamol (fever reducing drug), and diclofenac (pain killer) have gone up nearly 10% every year in last one decade. This is even higher than the inflation and wage increase of common public. That means we need to pay more for our medicines even if our income does not increase. Why does it happen and what are the remedies?

Like other consumer products, the price of medicines too depends on raw material cost, conversion cost (making into medicine for use), packaging cost, taxes and duties, marketing cost and profit to be made. But the medicines differ from other consumer products at least in two ways. Medicines are life saving and they improve or promote or maintain our health. There is no choice for consumers to buy. It is the doctor who decides or the chemist decides what the consumers buy. Rarely the consumer exerts his or her choice. It is who decides does not pay and who pays has no choice. How interesting!

In developed countries the health care cost inclusive of the cost of medicines is covered under insurance or social security system. But in a country like ours these schemes are either non-existing or not popular. People pay from their pocket. In order to protect the interest of common public, the government of India introduced drug price control order as early as 1970 to control the prices of all medicines. Unfortunately in the name liberalization and promoting the growth of pharmaceutical industries, the drug price control order is subsequently liberalized. It has been claimed that the growth of pharmaceutical industries with various brands available in the market will stabilize price on its own. It happens in other consumer goods where competition stabilizes the market price. But not in medicines! The same media which reported the 10% increase in medicine prices too reported that there is just 1% increase in prices of 15 medicines which are under drug price control mechanism during the same period of observation.

To save on medicines, ask for generics or least cost trusted brands.

The drug policy should ideally be designed or formulated taking health as main consideration. But unfortunately it often gets sidelined and the industries interest gets priority. The drug policy is the statement and guiding force for the government to initiate measure to solve medicine related issues including consumers' interest. The draft policy, pharmaceutical policy 2006, is yet to take a full shape because of several objections. The policy tried to make a balance of health aspects and consumers' interest on one side and the commercial interest on the other side. It is unfortunate that the responsibility of drafting and implementing the drug policy lies with the ministry of chemicals and fertilizers, but not on with the ministry of health.

The Indian medicine market is flooded with large number of formulations and drugs and many of which are unnecessary, irrational and harmful. The World Health Organization suggested the concept of essential drugs. These are medicines that satisfy the priority health needs of the population. These should be available all the time at an affordable rate and should be of assured quality. It is necessary that the government of India must take steps to control the prices of at least all the medicines which are covered under Essential Medicine List. The WHO revises this list every alternate year. Some of the state governments revise the list periodically. But the list of government of India is not regularly up dated. The last revision was on 2015.

The prices of medicines in the market vary widely. There are variations even among the leading brands. The generics are cheaper. Often a company has both brand and generic version of same medicine. Brands are costlier because lot of money is spent on promoting and building the image. In absence of adverse quality testing report, brands and generics are equal for all purpose.

General guidelines for the consumers to tackle this price rise situation:

- Ask for cheaper brand (of course to which you can trust).
- Use generics from reputed manufacturer.
- Check the price while buying medicines. Now there is no local tax. The maximum retail price is inclusive of all taxes. It is net price.
- Avail the discount offered by many chain pharmacies. Often their storage practice of medicines is better. They have temperature controlled condition for medicine storage.
- Try to impress the policy makers on a need of pro people drug policy. The citizens' demand will force the government to act.

[Update: The Government of India notified new price regulation for all essential medicines including cancer medicines. It has brought down the prices of 348 essential medicines. The regulation puts a cap on the prices of other medicines too: not to allow the increase in price beyond 10% per annum]

CHAPTER 8

Expiry Date of Medicines

(a) Expiry Date of Medicines

One of the most important things a consumer must look into while buying or using medicine is expiry date printed on the package and label of the product. Expiry date means the date after which the medicine is not fit for use. Sometimes, in place of expiry date the medicines are labelled with "Do not use after ---". The manufacturing company based on experiments fixes this expiry date and this is valid for original container, in which medicine is supplied, packaged and recommended storage conditions.

Like other consumable articles medicine too starts degrading moment it is made. Heat (temperature), light and moisture are the main factors responsible for drug degradation. It is important to maintain the recommended storage condition throughout the logistics. Drug decomposition (retention of potency) is not the only criterion that decides expiry date. The degraded product may be toxic. A physical change too can affect expiry date. A medicine needs to be physically, chemically, therapeutically and toxicologically stable.

Do not buy medicines close to the expiry date.
Do not use any medicine after expiry date.

The time period between the manufacturing date to the expiry date is called shelf life. In order to have reasonable shelf life for marketing a product, the manufacturing company, sometimes, adds overages (excess quantity) of active or medicinal ingredient. The purpose of adding overages is to maintain the minimum standard required (potency) till the expiry date.

In general, medicines available in the solid forms have better stability than the corresponding liquid forms. It is, sometimes, possible to recognize the degradation by noticing physical changes such as change in colour, odour or appearance. Aspirin tablets develop vinegar odour on degradation is an example.

A medicine, which was useful just on the last day of the month, is suddenly not useful next day. It sounds unbelievable. In fact there is no sudden death as it happens in biological or living system. But it is necessary to give a date beyond which medicine is not to be used, failing which they will be sold or made available for use without time limit causing safety threat to the users.

As our logistics and retail drug outlets are often not well equipped for appropriate storage conditions, the medicine may expire well before the expiry date printed on the label. It is preferable to avoid buying medicines nearing expiry date.

Do not use medicines after the expiry date. Throw away the unused or left over medicines after this date.

(b) Do Really Medicines Expire?

A casual look at the label of any medicine gives us the date of manufacturing and the date of expiry of the medicine. This is a legal requirement for the manufacturers to mention them on the label. Though these two are dates, they are mentioned as month and year. While the date of manufacturing may not be of interest to the medicine users, the date of expiry is always a concern for consumers.

The month written in expiry date indicates the last day of the month. A medicine with expiry date of March 2012 is legally permissible to sell and use till 31 March 2012. The question often raised "What happened to the medicine?" The medicine was effective and usable yesterday (31 March 2012), but not usable on 1 April 2012. Whether the medicines have similar to biological death!!This present article deals with these issues.

It is the responsibility of the manufacturers to ensure that the medicines are safe and effective during the entire shelf life of the products. To become effective, it is necessary to retain potency of the medicines. The shelf life of the medicinal products is determined based on scientific experimentation conducted by the manufacturers and they fix the date. This date is valid if the products are stored at recommended storage conditions. The validity of no use if not stored properly.

The current Indian Pharmacopoeia, the book of standards for medicines, specifies the storage conditions as store in a dry, well ventilated place at temperature not exceeding 30°C; store in a refrigerator (2 to 8 °C), do not freeze; store in a freezer (- 2°C to - 18°C) and store in a deep freezer (below -18°C). The temperature, humidity and light are the most detrimental factors that influence the potency of medicines during shelf life. The manufacturers usually have protective packing to prevent loss of potency due to exposure to high humidity or ultra violet light. The manufacturers have no mechanism to have control over the exposure of medicine to adversely affecting either high or low temperature. The rate of drug degradation doubles for every 10°C rise in temperature. During the distribution cycle of medicines including the chemists' shelf, the medicines get exposed to much higher temperature than the maximum recommended 30°C. We have air conditioned textile show room, shoes store etc. but no medical store! A tragedy! Neither the drugs control authority nor do chemists look this issue of preserving potency over the entire shelf life of the product. The medicines expire well before the expiry date. But we continue using.

In fact, there is nothing like biological deaths to medicines. Assuming up to the loss of 10% potency, the medicines would remain effective, the expiry date is fixed. At the last date of shelf life the medicines must have at least 90% of the labeled potency [this is a general requirement; it may vary with some medicines]. The loss of potency occurs over a period of time and is mostly dependent on storage temperature. To substantiate further, one should look into the warehouses constructed in almost every district of Tamil Nadu and Kerala where the appropriate storage conditioned are maintained including complete air conditioning of the warehouse to preserve the potency of the medicines supplied through government run health facilities.

In addition to potency, the safety of the medicines beyond expiry date is a matter of concern. There are few medicines which are more toxic on degradation than the original. The Tetracycline decomposes to epianhydrotetracycline that causes renal tubular damage. Chloroquine can produce toxic reactions attribute to photochemical degradation. Chlordiazepoxide and nitrazepamare known to cause phototoxicity. Infusion of degraded Penicillin G causes sensitization of lymphocytes and formation of antipenicilloyl antibodies.

Even the physical integrity of the product is temperature sensitive. The ointment and suppositories melt at temperature as high as 40°C. Low temperature is also troublesome for some medicines. Many insulin products are to be kept in refrigerator, but not to be frozen. On freezing it loses the desired activity. Similarly heparin becomes unstable if frozen. It is the responsibility of the manufacturers and the distributors to ensure the physical, chemical, therapeutic and toxicological stability of the medicines in the interest of public health.

Rationally speaking the drug product is suitable for use even after the expiry date if properly stored. But the ethical and legal dilemma remains whether to use the expired product or not!

CHAPTER 9

Storing Medicines at Home

Safe and effective use of medicine is the motto of every drug therapy decision. The safety and effectiveness of medicines very often depend on " how are they stored or kept at home?" Storing appropriately can prevent medicine mishap and preserve their quality. The life of medicines as mentioned as expiry date depends on storage conditions. If not stored appropriately, the medicines may expire well before the expiry date.

A child has been watching mother taking colored pills every day. One day while mother is away, he started exploring them and found them to be like candy. He swallowed few pills. The mother on return found the child to be in serious condition. This is the story of sugar coated iron tablets. The accidental use of medicine by children can be disastrous. It is essential that all medicines must be kept out of sight and reach of children preferably in a locked cabinet.

Heat and moisture have damaging effect on the quality of medicines. They need to be protected from high temperature and humidity. Kitchen and bathroom are hot and humid places. Medicines are never to be kept in these places. Some medicines require storage in controlled temperature like keeping in a refrigerator where temperature is usually maintained between 2-8°C. Unless advised medicines are never be kept in refrigerator.

Heat, light and moisture are degrading factors for medicines. Always keep medicines away from reach of children.

Some medicines are affected by UV light. Sunlight should never be allowed to fall on these medicines. These medicines are normally packaged in amber colored bottle and an outer box is used for providing further protection. The medicines must be kept in the outer box after use.

The instruction for storage requirement is written on the label. The following are few examples: Store in a cool dry place; store in a cold place; protect from light; do not store at temperature exceeding 25 °C. The cold place means temperature between 2-8 °C, and cool place means a place where temperature is maintained at 8-25 °C (air conditioned).

Below are the few tips for proper storing of medicines:

- Keep away from the reach of children.
- Do not keep in hot place like kitchen and humid place like bathrooms.
- Preferably keep in AC room if available.
- Do not keep them in your car for long period.
- Keep in refrigerator, if recommended only.
- Protect the medicines from direct exposure of sunlight.
- Keep medicines separately for different persons.
- Keep medicines in their original containers.
- Always return medicines to the storage place after use even if you require them again.

Safe guard your family against medicines misuse and abuse by keeping all medicines in a safe place.

CHAPTER 10

Laws and Regulations Governing Medicines

Medicines are perhaps the greatest weapon of mankind to fight disease and death. They save lives, restore health, prevent diseases and stop epidemics. In order to perform the above functions, they must be safe, effective and be of good quality and used appropriately. To assure the above attributes, the government of India regulates imports, manufacturing and sale of medicines. Medicines regulation is a public health and social welfare measure of central and state governments.

In the present article various laws governing the different aspects of medicines control is briefly narrated. This would make the consumers or readers aware of the various provisions so that they can exercise their rights and take or initiate appropriate measures in public interest to safe guard individual and public health. The discussion is not exhaustive; the readers are advised to go through the details of the Act for more information.

The medicine control in India was enforced since pre independent era through a colonial legislation, the Drugs Act 1940. Since then many amendments to the Act were made: Cosmetics and medicines of other systems of medicines like Ayurvedic, Unanai and Sidha and Homeopathy are brought under this legislation. In the present form this legislation is known as Drugs and Cosmetics Act 1940 and the Rules 1945. Under the Act the government of India through Central Drug Standard Control Organization and the state governments through Directorate of Drugs Control (in some states Food and Drugs Administration) control the various operations: import, manufacture, distribution and sale of medicines. Drugs Controller General (India) and the State Drugs Controller are the chief executive and administrative authorities for implementation of various provisions of the Act. Drugs Inspectors are the officers at the lowest level of drug regulation operating at usually district level.

The government of India implemented good manufacturing practice (GMP) guidelines in order to assure manufacturing of quality medicines only. The manufacturers must follow these GMP specifications. Import, manufacturing and sale of medicines are permitted under license only. Sale of medicines is usually through a retail pharmacy or drug store, which engages the service of a registered pharmacist.

Though Drugs and Cosmetics Act is referred as a live saving statute, it is not amended as per social need. Some recommendations (Mashelkar Committee) are pending before the central government for adoption. Once they are adopted, the drugs control system in the country would be further strengthened.

Narcotic Drugs and Psychotropic Substance Act 1985 is another piece of progressive legislation which controls the operations relating to addiction forming and mood (behavior) changing substances. Such substances have more stringent control, as they are likely to be misused or abused. There are stringent punishment provisions for indulging in illegal activities relating to these drugs and substances.

Medicines are regulated substances. They are regulated at all levels from manufacturing to use including their pricing.

Though other system of medicines are in practice in our country, the allopathic qualified doctor can not practice (prescribe) medicines of other systems and the vice versa. The medicines price is too controlled by the central government in order to make them affordable through Drugs Price Control order 1995. The original drugs price control order is much diluted and at present only few medicines are under price control mechanism. The government must make provision for controlling all essential medicines in order to make them affordable. The country has very poor drug accessibility: just one third of population against the world average of two third.

Through Drugs and Magic Remedies Act 1954, the unethical and misleading advertisements relating drugs and drug treatment are prohibited to protect the innocent publics from getting exploited and to prevent self medication.

A milestone in the socio economic legislation is Consumer Protection Act 1985. Under the act consumer (or a Patient) can seek compensation if he or she suffers from the use of wrong medicines or counterfeit or poor quality of medicines. The consumer has the right to know about his or her medicines from both the prescribing doctor and dispensing pharmacist both at hospital and private practice.

Though we have good regulations that control the availability of safe, effective and quality medicines for the countrymen, they are poorly implemented. The consumers and the community must demand the effective regulations. Here are few tips:

- Insist on safe medicines. The medicines, which are banned in other countries, should also be banned.
- Insist on getting information about medicines you buy and keep the receipt of medicines purchased.
- Complain to the government agencies or authorities if you come across illegal activities relating medicines.

Your active participation and involvement can make life better for you and others.

CHAPTER 11

Rational use of Medicines

Medicines are perhaps the most important weapon of mankind to fight disease and illness. But they are two ways weapons. No medicine is safe and does only good thing without an element of risk. It is the benefit-risk ratio that counts. They are costly too. Though accessibility of medicines is a human right, two third of India's population does not have access to such medicines against the world's average of one –third. Promoting rational use of medicines is a recommended strategy for improving accessibility and promoting safe and effective use of medicines.

World Health Organization defines rational use of medicines "Patients receive medications appropriate to their clinical needs, in doses that meet their own requirements, for an adequate period of time, and at the lowest cost to them and their community". There are many examples in day-to-day medicine use. Some of them are: use of too many medicines per patient; inappropriate use of antimicrobials, often in inadequate doses, for non bacterial infections; overuse of injections, when oral preparations are more effective; inappropriate self medication, especially with prescription only medicines. Inappropriate dosage may cause serious problem including leading to mortality in childhood diseases and in treatment of chronic conditions like diabetes, hypertension etc. Overuse of medicines wastes our resources as we pay for it. Overuse and inappropriate use of antimicrobials leads to increased antimicrobial resistance. Overuse especially use of non-sterile injection sets increases the risk of contamination of hepatitis, HIV etc.

Rational Medicine use means right medicine:

- For the right person;
- For the right illness;
- At the right time;
- In the right dose;
- For the right length of time; and
- At the right price

There are several reasons of irrational medicine use: lack of knowledge, skills, or independent information, unrestricted availability of medicines, unethical and inappropriate medicine promotion and profit motive from selling medicines.

The patients need access to accurate and understandable information about potential benefits and risks of medicine in general; how do they act in the body; the limitations of drug therapy and other treatment options. The present day consumers are no longer passive medicine users. They must take part as informed partner in drug therapy decision making and subsequent drug use. People frequently waste money on medicines. Often they are not aware that cheaper generic equivalents are available in the market. There are even significant variations in prices among the branded products of same medicine. Costlier medicines are better is not always true.

Take or Use medicines only when required. Learn about your medicines – More you know better they work.

To ensure that you use medicine in the right way, always ask your doctor or pharmacist the following questions:

- What is the name of the medicine and what it is supposed to do?
- When and how often should be taken?
- Can it be taken along with other medicines?
- Are there any side effects?
- Do I continue my normal activity after taking the medicine?
- Are there some foods to be avoided? Is it to be taken before or after food?

- Should I continue to take until it is finished or stop when I feel better?
- What shall I do if I miss a dose?
- How much does it cost? Are there cheaper ones?

The doctors and pharmacists are professionally responsible even with their all busy schedule for providing guidance and counseling on medicines they prescribe, advise or dispense. It is patients' duty and rights to know about the medicines they are going use from them. Be careful about the commercial drug promotions, often they are misleading. Remember the medicines are essential to be used appropriately and safely for your benefit and safety and should be used only when needed.

(Courtesy: ABC of Rational Use of Medicines, Health Action International, Africa)

CHAPTER 12

How do Medicines Work

The different medicines work different ways. Some medicines provide immediate relief while others require prolonged use to exert significant benefits. In this article, the simplified mechanisms are described through which the medicines exert their effects.

Most medicines exert their action after entering into body system through various means. The medicines enter into blood after being swallowed, injected, or absorbed through skin and carried throughout the body and reach the target site, the place for medicines to act. At the target site medicine interact with the cellular components called receptors. The medicine-receptor interaction is specific. In this way the medicines modify the biochemical or metabolic process of body's cells or enzyme systems to change the course of a disease process. Morphine provides pain-relieving action through interacting with the receptors in the brain. Anti-asthma medicine like theophylline and salbutamol too work by dilating the bronchial muscles. Medicine, lovastatin, used to treat people of high blood cholesterol level, act by interacting with enzyme system which is critical in body's production of cholesterol. Cimetidine, ranitidine like medicines, used to treat gastric ulcers act, by reducing the acid secretion by blocking the acid secreting cells.

Another important categories of medicines known as antibiotics (antimicrobial agents) exert their effects by modifying the metabolic activity of invaded pathogenic microorganisms. The disease conditions produced by these microbes are called infections and accordingly such medicines are known as anti-infective. These categories medicines on absorption into the system interfere with microbes' growth or kill them. Penicillin, erythromycin, tetracycline, norfloxacin etc. come under this category.

A small number of medicines act by chemical reaction with gastric hydrochloric acid. They reduce the excessive acidity by neutralizing the acid in the stomach and hence called gastric antacids. These types of medicines are not required to be absorbed into the system and get excreted through feces. Aluminium hydroxide, magnesium hydroxide, magnesium trisilicate come under this category of medicines.

The medicines act on body's cells or enzyme systems to change the course of a disease process.

Some medicines exert their effects through physical action. The simple non-medicated ointments or creams provide protective action on application over skin. The liquid paraffin causes smooth passage of stool through its lubricating effect in the intestinal wall.

The medicines which work either by interacting with the receptors or enzyme system or invading microorganisms need to have at least a minimum concentration in blood in order to exert therapeutic response. Below this concentration they would not be effective. This minimum concentration maintenance is dependent on dosage regimen. The number of units like tablets to be taken and at what interval constitutes the dosage regimen. The patients need to adhere this dosage schedule as prescribed in order to derive maximum benefits from medicines' use failing which there is possibility that they may not get any relief or expose themselves to toxic effects of overdosing.

The medicines that enter into blood, gets distributed to various tissues including target site. They too undergo metabolism and elimination. All these process occur simultaneously. Metabolism and elimination are medicine removal process from the body. The liver and kidney are main metabolizing and eliminating organ respectively. Their function determines how frequently the medicine needs to be taken. That is why if these organs do not function normally, the different dosage regimen is fixed in such condition. If the patients know of their liver or kidney problem, they need to inform the physicians so that the correct dosage regimen of appropriate medicines is prescribed to them.

CHAPTER 13

Fate of Medicines in the Body (How does Body Handle Medicines?)

Though medicines are delivered into our body by many ways, they need to enter the blood stream (called absorption) so that they can be carried into the place of action (receptors). There are few exceptions like gastric antacids, which are not meant for entry into blood. Once they entered blood, along with the blood they gets distributed into other organs and tissues including fluids. Different medicines depending on their properties get access to different places in the body to different extent. Thus all organs and tissues are exposed to the beneficial and ill effects of medicines. While ideally, it is necessary that the medicines should reach the site of action in adequate quantity, exposure to other places in the body should be avoided, but practically, rarely it is feasible.

On entry into blood, the body starts processing them so that they can be easily eliminated or excreted. Our body system treats them as foreign objects. Two of our vital organs Liver and Kidneys work through a series of process for this purpose. Liver with the help of its enzymes breaks down the medicines to make them more favourable for elimination by kidneys. This conversion process is known as metabolism or biodegradation (also called detoxification). The products of metabolism are metabolites and as they are more water soluble, easily get removed by kidneys. The metabolites are sometimes even medicinally active and provide therapeutic action. On rare occasions the medicines by pass liver and excreted in-tact un-metabolised.

The medicine metabolism is different in different persons and is influenced by age, race and presence of other drugs. Metabolising enzyme systems are partially developed at birth. As newborns have difficulty in metabolising many drugs, the dose of medicines is proportionally lower based on body weight basis, the way dose is usually determined. But the children require proportionately higher dose. The elderly too have problems of reduced enzymatic activity and there is a need for reduced dose.

Genetic differences among people too affect metabolism. Some people metabolise them slowly while others do it faster. Thus the medicines will either stay longer or shorter period of time in the body depending on slow and first metabolism. This genetic difference is particularly common in certain ethnic groups and races.

Some medicines alter the liver enzyme systems responsible for medicine metabolism: both inactivation and stimulation happens. When one medicine inactivates the metabolising enzyme responsible for metabolising another medicine, the concentration of the latter medicine increases and stays longer period of time in the body. When enzyme system is stimulated, the drug stay in system becomes shorter. It gets quickly eliminated. In both situations dose adjustment is necessary. If phenobarbitone (sedative) is administered together with warfarin (for preventing blood clotting), the latter becomes less effective as its metabolism is increased in presence of the former. In this situation, there may be need of increasing the dose of warfarin. But if the phenobarbitone is later withdrawn and the dose of warfarin is not reduced, it could lead to potentially serious situation. Cigarette smoking too increases the enzyme activity of liver.

During liver and kidney problems, dose adjustment may be necessary. Tell your problems to doctors.

The drug metabolism is also disturbed in liver disease, though extent of problem is difficult to ascertain.

Kidneys filter the drugs or metabolites from the blood and excrete them into urine. The water-soluble materials are easily filtered. The kidneys ability to excrete drugs depends on several factors like acidity of urine, urine flow and the conditions of kidneys. The kidney function normally decreases with advancement of age. Many diseases like blood pressure, diabetes and kidney infection can impair kidney functions. The impaired kidney function results in increased duration of medicines' stay in the body and thus necessitate the need of dose reduction. As the extent of kidney functioning is measurable (unlike liver function), the dose can be optimised (exactly adjusted) based on individual requirement. The creatinine clearance is a measure of kidney function.

Small amounts of medicines are also excreted in saliva, breast milk, bile, sweat and even exhaled air.

As body needs to do a lot of exercises to process the medicines to eliminate them, it is not advisable to take medicines when they are really not wanted. To promote safe and effective medication here are few tips:

Tell your doctor if you have liver or kidney problem. Dose adjustment may be necessary. Certain medicines need to avoided as they are either toxic or further damage these organs.

Avoid unnecessary medications as they burden your vital organs like liver and kidneys.

Self-medications could be harmful if you are not knowledgeable.

CHAPTER 14

Safety of Medicines (How do you Protect Yourself?)

The medicines are perhaps the greatest weapon of mankind to fight diseases and illness. The medicines are subjected to stringent experimental protocol for establishing the efficacy and safety before being allowed for mass use. However, no short and limited study (pre-marketing trial) can completely evaluate the benefit and risk involved in a medicine use. A medicine found for one ailment is later discovered to have other usefulness. A classic example is aspirin. It was initially discovered as pain and fever relieving substance and now finds wide use as treatment for various heart problems. Similarly many undetected risks are discovered later.

It is quoted "No medicine is 100% safe for all people in all circumstances". All medicines have one or other side effects. They are reported during clinical evaluation of medicines before approval for mass use. Dreams, reduced menstruation, dry mouth, skin rash, headache, diarrhoea, nausea etc., are just few examples and usually they are not serious. However, some medicines have unexpected side effects called adverse drug reactions which may be serious or life threatening. These effects are unusual and difficult to observe especially during pre-marketing trial. They are usually detected when medicines are in wide use in large populations. In a study, safety is always judged in relation to effectiveness or usefulness of medicine.

No medicine is absolutely safe. Report the experienced adverse reaction to your doctor or pharmacist.

The worst form of adverse drug reaction was reported after use of so called safe pill for sleeping disorder, thalidomide. The use of this by pregnant ladies has resulted in severely deformed infants in early 1960s in several countries. Thalidomide was immediately banned. This terrible lesson has made the whole world to continue monitoring the safety of medicines during their wider use, a study called post-marketing surveillance. Such study has resulted in ensuring safer medicines for the patients. A recent example is withdrawal of rofecoxib, a pain relieving substance, from US market and banning the same in our country.

With support of international agencies, the government of India has recently launched a nationwide adverse drug reaction monitoring, termed as pharmacovigilance programme. To begin with, the health care professionals are encouraged to report any adverse reaction they encounter during their practice. But it is the patient who only knows the actual benefit and harm of a medicine taken. Observation and report made by a health professional is just an interpretation of a description originally provided by the patient. Patients who suspect that they have been affected by an adverse drug reaction are normally encouraged to report their doctor or pharmacist, who would in turn report the same to safety monitoring center, currently called pharmacovigilance center.

Direct advertisement of both prescription and non-prescription medicines to the consumers, and the flooded information in net have resulted in increasing self-medication. As these adverse drug reactions are unexpected and unusual, the patients or consumers need to be vigilant and they must report back their experience to the doctor or pharmacist. Even they have the liberty to directly report to the southern regional center located at JIPMER, Pondicherry; though there are many peripheral centers.

Another important area that requires consumers' attention is a myth "Natural means safe. The herbal and traditional medicines are absolutely safe". The truth is different. They are toxic too. Patients are required to be equally vigilant while using herbal or similar medicines.

The report of adverse drug reaction by health care professionals and the patients will go in a long way formulating better policies with a view to reducing patients' risk and improving patients' safety.

As a precautionary measure to harvest the maximum benefit from medicine use with a minimum risk, the patient needs to:

- Procure right medicines as prescribed.
- Know medicine use and follow the instructions given.
- Inform the doctor or pharmacist of any medicine including OTC and herbals currently one is using.
- Report any different effects they observe or experience.

CHAPTER 15

Medicines can be Toxic Too

"I saw my friend's wife dead after using the inhaler for asthma and hence I am afraid of using it" says a reader from Kerala, a chronic asthma patient. He continues narrating "as she developed an attack of asthma in night, continued using it repeatedly since she did not get relief after the recommended dose".

The reader is actually confused. The benefits of using medicines are well known but the toxicity (sometimes called side effects, adverse effects etc.) of them is little known. No medicine is 100 % safe to all individuals in all circumstances. Usually benefits outweigh the risks in medicine and medicine related therapy. Though the medicines have undergone a well-defined testing procedure both at pre-clinical (testing on animals) and clinical (testing on human beings) testing stages for establishing the safety and efficacy, still none is completely free from toxicity. In this particular case there could be another possibility, which cannot be ruled out. The inhaler could be empty and the patient continued using it ignorantly. In another episode of the column, we shall discuss the appropriate use of these inhalers.

The toxicity of pressurized inhalers causing deaths in young asthmatics was first reported as early as in 1960. The prestigious British Medical Journal in 1967 reported "patients with asthma were killing themselves by excessive use of metered aerosols (inhalers)". Toxicity of thalidomide (used as sleeping tablets) during pregnancy causing serious birth defects and sulphanilamide elixir (prepared with toxic solvent, diethylene glycol) causing deaths of many children are well known in the history of medicine use. Some people, though limited in number, may be allergic to certain medicines or components of medicines. Penicillin injection can cause serious life threatening situation, anaphylactic shock, in small number of peoples. The injection is tested with a test dose before administering the injection to avoid the risk.

The doctors, health care professionals often make mistakes causing medication error. There are evidences that excessive and inappropriate prescription of medicines contributes substantially to the occurrence of adverse drug reactions. Patients too can make mistakes. Taking many medicines or receiving treatment from more than one source can contribute significantly to causing medicine related problems, particularly harmful interactions.

It is not that the toxicity of medicines is always serious. Most often they are tolerable. The toxicity may result from either use of usual dose or from excessive dose. They are not restricted to prescription medicines alone, even the over the counter medicines too are associated with problems. The medicines of other system of medicines are not exceptional. Heavy metal toxicity of some herbal products has been recently reported.

No medicine is 100% safe to all individuals at all circumstances. Use medicines only when required.

Assessment or monitoring of toxicity of medicines during use (post marketing surveillance) is an important requirement for marketing license. Though such programmes were in existence in many countries, this is a new initiative in our country. The government of India has launched National Pharmacovigilance Programme with several centers across the country for monitoring the safety of medicines. The Pharmacovigilance programme identifies the medicines causing serious harm and initiate action before widespread damage occurs. A recent example is withdrawal of valdecoxib, an anti-inflammatory agent, from the world market. The doctors, health care professionals and patients should make it a point to report any toxicity event that they notice during use of medicines to the nearest centre or to the central drug standard control organization of government of India (details can be found at www.cdsco.nic.in) to improve safety data base of medicines.

Here are few general guidelines for the patients to follow to ensure safe use of medicines:

- Use medicines as recommended. Adhere to dosage schedule (dose and timing). Avoid excessive dose.
- Learn the proper use of medicines either from your doctor or pharmacist.

- Consult your doctor, if you do not get the desired relief of your symptoms or illness even after using medicines.
- Avoid self-medication, unless you are thorough with disease and medicines. Self-medication can not only be misleading but could be dangerous too.
- Avoid use of prescription medicines without doctor's advice.
- If you experience any toxicity or unusual effects during medicine's use, immediately report to your doctor or pharmacist.
- To know more on the medicines prescribed or using, ask for package inserts to your pharmacist. Pharmaceutical companies usually supply them.

CHAPTER 16

Adherence to Medications

It is often found that the patients do not (or, fail to) follow the dosage schedule specified or prescribed for them. This results in not getting relief of illness as medicines become ineffective. It leads to a lot of confusion even doubting the authenticity or quality of medicines.

The extent to which the patients follow the instruction of doctors on medicine use is called adherence, or simply compliance. There are many reasons why patients sometimes fail to or do not follow the dosage schedule. Dosage schedule means the numbers of dose, number of times per day and the total period of use. The important reasons for this non-adherence are: dosage schedule is too complex and not understood, especially when several medicines are prescribed together; difficulty in keeping the dosage schedule because of life style; lack of confidence in either doctor or medicines; experience of undesired effects; lack of money to buy the complete course; and the influence of incorrect and conflicting information from patient's family, friend or relative. Patients on short-term medication have better adherence rate than those on long-term therapy.

Patients need to adhere to the dosage schedule in order to derive maximum benefit from the use of medicines.

The non-adherence can worsen the quality of life. Missed dose of glaucoma medicine may lead to optic nerve damage and blindness; missed dose of heart medicine may lead to erratic heart rhythm. The non-adherence is not only the problem of individual patient but is a threat to the community, when anti-microbial agents (including antibiotics) are not properly used. These medicines are germ-killing agents. They provide relief or cure from infectious diseases caused by germs. The non-adherence of anti-microbial drugs schedule leads to sub therapeutic exposure of these medicines. The exposure to low dose level not only causes the drug to become ineffective at the moment, but also may become ineffective permanently due to development of resistance. In fact, the anti-microbial resistance is a global threat.

One of the greatest problems encountered is ineffective tuberculosis treatment strategy because of poor adherence. The tuberculosis treatment requires prolonged treatment with several medicines. On use of medicines, the patients feel better and get a false impression that they are cured of illness. They do not complete the full course of medicines. That is why, worldwide a new strategy is introduced, called DOTS (directly observed treatment short course), to improve patients' adherence to TB dosage schedule. In this programme another person ensures that the patient is taking his medicines as per schedule.

Even the best treatment plan will fail if not followed properly. In order to derive the maximum benefits from medicines use, the patients need to adhere the treatment schedule. Study have shown that the participation of patients with doctors in therapeutic decision making process of his treatment improve adherence. In order to comply with required dosage schedule of medicines the patients should:

- Discuss with the doctors on medicine treatment plan.
- Clearly understand the dosage schedule of all the medicines prescribed.
- Ask for written instruction for medicines use schedule either from doctor or pharmacist who gives you the medicines.
- Inform the doctor about the unwanted or unexpected effects experienced, before adjusting the dose or stopping treatment. The doctor can make appropriate adjustment of dose or change the medicine.
- Inform the doctor if you have difficulty in frequently taking medicines either because of forgetfulness or due to inconvenience. The doctor may prescribe long acting medicines, which are required to be taken less frequently, sometimes, even just once a day. Such long acting medicines improve adherence.

CHAPTER 17

Missing a Dose (If you Miss a Dose ----)

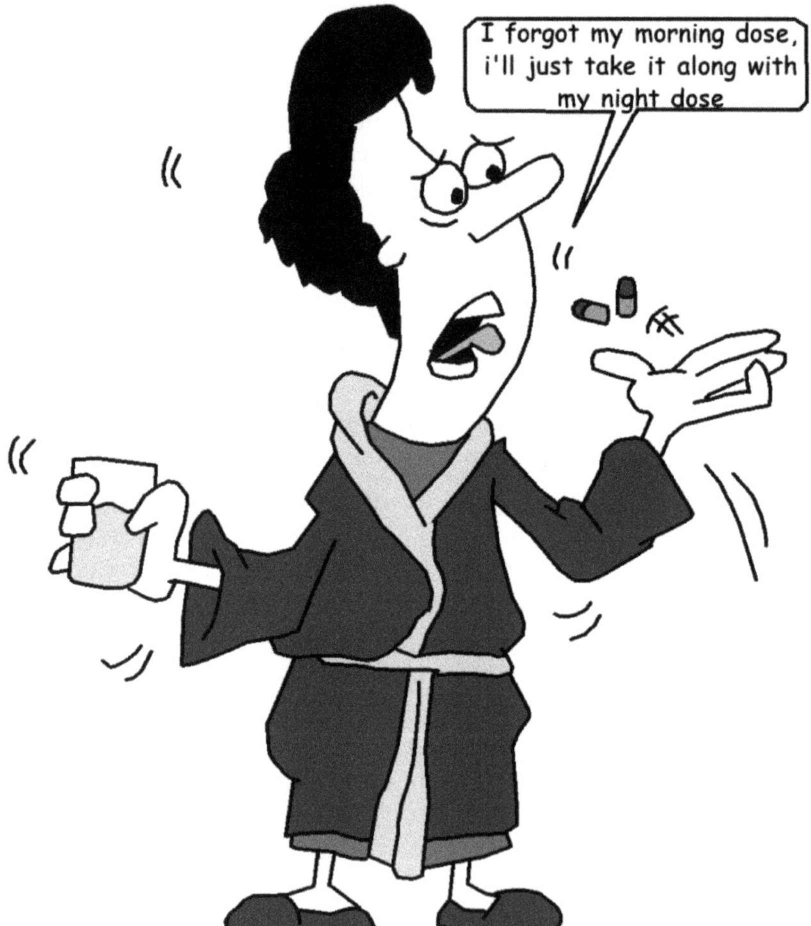
I forgot my morning dose, i'll just take it along with my night dose

"Doubling the dose can be dangerous, Follow doctor's or pharmacist advice"

"More than 50% of patients fail to take the medicines correctly," a WHO report says. There are many reasons for this non-compliance. Some of them are: not understanding or misinterpreting the medication instruction; forgetting to take medicines; experiencing adverse effects of medicines; not believing that the medicines can help; mistakenly believing that the illness has been treated successfully; finding difficult to take like swallowing tablets, self injecting insulin and worrying about expenses. However, forgetfulness is one of the main causes and very often it is not deliberate. Even the best drug treatment plan may fail if not properly followed.

The dose and dosage regimens (how many times to be taken or used per day), advised for the patients, are essential to maintain a therapeutic level of medicines in the blood. The desired medicine's level is usually maintained in such a way that it is more than the minimum effective concentration and below the toxic concentration. Less concentration will result in no effects and high concentrations would cause toxic effects.

Very often the patients forget to take medicines and miss a dose. They do not know what to do. The effect of missed dose is different in different medicines. It depends on clinical condition of the patients and medicines prescribed or advised. The patients suffering from illness (epilepsy, blood clotting in the system) where a constant medicines' level is essential are very vulnerable for significant effects of missed dose. The narrow therapeutic indexed medicines too have significant problems if dose is missed. A narrow therapeutic index means a small increase or decrease in concentration may cause toxic effects or no effects respectively. On the other hand, for most patients missing dose occasionally is of little significance.

Even the best drug treatment plan may fail if not properly followed. Do not double your dose at any time.

The missing doses of oral contraceptives have significance bearings and there is a risk of unwanted pregnancy. The combined pills are advised to take for 21 consecutive days starting on 5th day of menstrual cycle followed by a break of 7 days during which menstruation occurs. However to improve compliance the pills are made available as package of 28 pills with 21 active pills and 7 belong to dummy or iron tablets. Mala – N and Mala – D fall in the category. If one or two tablets are missed from dummy tablets, no special precaution is necessary. The woman can continue taking remaining tablets as usual ignoring the missed tablet(s). If an active tablet is forgotten, take it as soon as it is remembered, within 12 hours of schedule time. Then continue taking next dose as usual. If there is delay of more than 12 hours after the time the tablet is normally taken, contraceptive effect is reduced. There is more risk of becoming pregnant, if the tablets are missed in first week or at the end of current pack (third week). Take missed tablet as soon as it is remembered, even if this means taking two tablets at a time. Continue taking daily tablet as usual and use additional contraceptive method for next seven days. For women who are under progestogen only pills (Minipills) are advised to continue additional contraceptive use for 14 days, if the dose is delayed by three hours or more.

Missed dose of glaucoma medicine can lead to optic nerve damage and blindness. Missed dose of heart medicine may lead to erratic heart rhythm and cardiac arrests. Missed dose of high blood pressure medicines may cause stroke. Missed dose of antibiotics may cause infections to flare up again and developing drug resistant bacteria. However in most of the cases, doubling of dose could be dangerous as there are chances of adverse effects of high concentration. If dose is missed and it is time for next dose (within two hours), it is preferable to skip off the dose and take the next dose as usual. Here are few guidelines:

- Ask your doctor or pharmacist what to do if a dose is missed. They would advise you appropriately.
- In case of oral contraceptives follow the guidelines discussed above and use additional contraceptive method.
- In all other cases, do not double the dose. If it is time for next dose, skip it off. Take the next dose in schedule time.
- Try to follow the dosage schedule as advised.

CHAPTER 18

Prescription and Non-prescription Medicines

The medicines are basically divided into two categories – prescription medicines and non-prescription medicines. Prescription medicines are those that could be habit forming, toxic and unsafe for use except under medical supervision. They need to be sold only the prescription of registered medical practitioners. All other medicines come under the non-prescription medicines, commonly called over the counter (OTC) medicines.

OTC is an American drug regulation terminology. In our country everything, both prescription and non-prescription medicine, is available over the counter endangering the public health. It is important and essential too, for the consumers to know the danger of using prescription medicines without medical advice and how to use OTC medicines safely.

No medicine is 100% safe. Every medicine is associated with some elements of risk. In order to get benefit from medicine use, it is required to take this risk. It is generally recognized that OTC medicines are safe, if appropriately used. The following household medicines come under this category: Aspirin tablets, pain balms, antacids, gripe waters for infants, nasal congestion inhalers, certain cough syrups/drops/lozenges, iron preparations, paracetamol preparations etc.

Paracetamol, a fever reducing and pain relieving medicine, is available in various brands and generic names with wide differences in their prices. This medicine is generally recognized as safe. A recently introduced warning label to advice the consumers not to exceed the recommended dose clearly demonstrate "how safe the drugs are". Do our consumers aware of the maximum daily dose or recommended dose? Is it written on the label of the product? The answer is obviously, no. We rarely find such information on the label. Even the liver toxicity of paracetamol becomes more acute, if the patient consumes alcohol or alcoholic drink.

Gastric antacids are seemed to be harmless if used alone. But when used along with certain other medicines like tetracycline, they interact and reduce the affect of the former. Iron preparations are likely to cause gastric irritation and are better tolerated if taken after meals. Aspirin tablets should not be used for children below 12 years. These are just few examples of problems associated with OTC medicines.

Do not self medicate with prescription medicines. Consult your doctor or pharmacist to know about your medicines.

Another potential danger is drug over lapping. Unless the label of medicines is properly checked, there is possibility of accidental over dosage. An example will clarify the situation. Paracetamol is a common ingredient in many cold and sinus products. If a person ignorantly takes a paracetamol tablet for headache along with a sinus product containing paracetamol is likely to overdose. This clearly indicates the necessity of medicine use information for the consumers. It is necessary that the consumers need to obtain necessary information like dose and how many times to take; what precaution to take while using the medicine; what are possible side effects etc.

People often neglect to inform their health care professionals that they have been using certain OTC medicines. As these medicines, sometimes, influence the affect of other prescription medicines, it is recommended that the patients disclose this to their doctors or pharmacists while seeking advice.

In order to safely use these OTC medicines, the consumers can look forward to their neighborhood pharmacists for necessary information, which can be obtained verbally or written form. The patient information leaflets (package inserts) are available for many medicines.

The following guidelines help consumers selecting most appropriate OTC medicine and to use them safely:

- Use OTC medicines for self care only for minor problems.
- Do not exceed recommended dose.
- Stop using the medicine if situation worsens or experience adverse effects.
- Select a product with fewest ingredients. As far as possible avoid medicines of multiple ingredients.

- Read the label of the medicines carefully to avoid duplication.
- Ask the pharmacists about the medicines you wish to know.

OTC medicines are primarily meant for occasional use and they are to be used only for few days for self-treatment. If necessary for regular use for long period, a medical advice is a must.

CHAPTER 19

Medicines for Children

The children are most loveable to all of us and at the same time they are very vulnerable too. About 13% of our country's population is between 0-6 years of age. Almost 40% of Indians are younger than 15 years of age. Though we often assume that they are miniature of adults, it is not true. There is wide variation in physiological functions between children and the adults. Many of the vital organs like liver and kidneys are not as developed as that of adults. They need very sensitive care and so as the types of medicines made available for their use.

While the medicines available in the market are well tested in clinical trials involving adults, the medicines are usually not tested in children. The medicinal therapies in children are just extension of results from the adults' trials. The world has not forgotten the medicinal disaster involving sulphanilamide elixir which killed more than 100 children in USA during 1930s. The sulphanilamide, a wonder antibacterial of the period, was made into a paediatric formulation (elixir) dissolving the sulphanilamide in diethylene glycol. Diethylene glycol is an extremely toxic solvent. This disaster was a good lesson and the USA government made the testing of the whole product mandatory for safety and efficacy (not just the active drug) before marketing approval. The similar incidents occurred in India too.

The children are classified by age as: Neonate – first four weeks of life (0-28 days); Infant – 1 to 12 months (1 month to 1 year); and child – 1 to 12 years. The neonatal period is very sensitive to medicine. During the period the body undergoes changes in enzyme activity. The immature liver and kidneys are inadequate with respect to detoxification and excretion. The new born and pre-maturely born and infants have immature liver and kidneys. A reduced capacity to detoxify and eliminate drugs can result in drug accumulation in the tissues to the toxic levels. The doses of children are often expressed in terms of mg per kg weight (mg/kg). Though most of the time this formula works out, but more appropriate method of calculating dose is based on body surface area. The body surface of the child can be calculated from the formula:

Body Surface Area (BSA) of the Child in square meter $\left(m^2\right) = \sqrt{\frac{\text{Height in cm} \times \text{weight in kg}}{3600}}$

$$\text{Child's dose} = \frac{\text{Adult dose}}{1.7\ m^2} \times \text{BSA of child}$$

The medicines for children are developed and manufactured using ingredients which are known to be safe for children. The alcoholic preparations used in adults may not be suitable for children. Alcohol can alter the liver function, cause gastric irritation and effect neurologic depression in neonate. The adult dosage forms may not be suitable for younger children. The use of these may expose the children for over dosing and unwanted side effects or under dosing without expected effects. The dosage forms are appropriate to deliver the recommended dose.

The children's medicine is made in a way that is designed to accurate administration of the dose to children of varying age and weight. At the same time its administration must be acceptable to the child and the adult care giver. In general, the medicines for the newborns are available as solutions, drops, nasal drops, suppositories, ointments and liquids for dermal application, injections, eye drops etc; for infants they are in the form of solutions, drops, emulsions, suspensions, nasal drops, suppositories, enemas, dermal ointments and liquids, injections, nebulizers, spacers, eye drops and ointments; the children are often given similar to the products available or used by adults.

Do not give medicines to children without medical advice. Use the medicinal spoon supplied along with medicine to measure the dose.

The tablets are sometimes recommended to be broken, crushed and given to the children after mixing with food or milk. Of the child does not like the taste of the medicine, he/she may even develop aversion to the milk. It is preferable not to mix medicine with milk. Problems of swallowing can be avoided by breaking the tablets into half or quarter (though not ideal), using dispersible or chewable or effervescent tablets. Seriously ill children may require injections. Orally administered medicines are preferable for long term use and rectal and transdermal products are too useful.

The care givers or parents are responsible for giving the medicines to the children. They should follow the following general guidelines while giving medicines to the children:

- Always consult your doctor preferably paediatrician before giving medicine to your child.
- Learn the dose and duration for the medicines prescribed for your child. Some medicines may be available in different strengths. For example, paracetamol syrup is available at 125 mg per 5 ml and 250 mg per 5 ml. If not careful, the dose may be doubled.
- Use the supplied dropper for measuring dose for infants.
- Adhere to the medication schedule as prescribed by the doctor.
- Use the same spoon (preferably measuring spoon supplied along with medicine) for measuring the dose. The capacities of the domestic spoons vary widely.
- Do not use the medicines prescribed for adults. Breaking the tablets are not advisable.
- Keep the medicines out of reach of children.

CHAPTER 20

Medicines for Elderly Persons

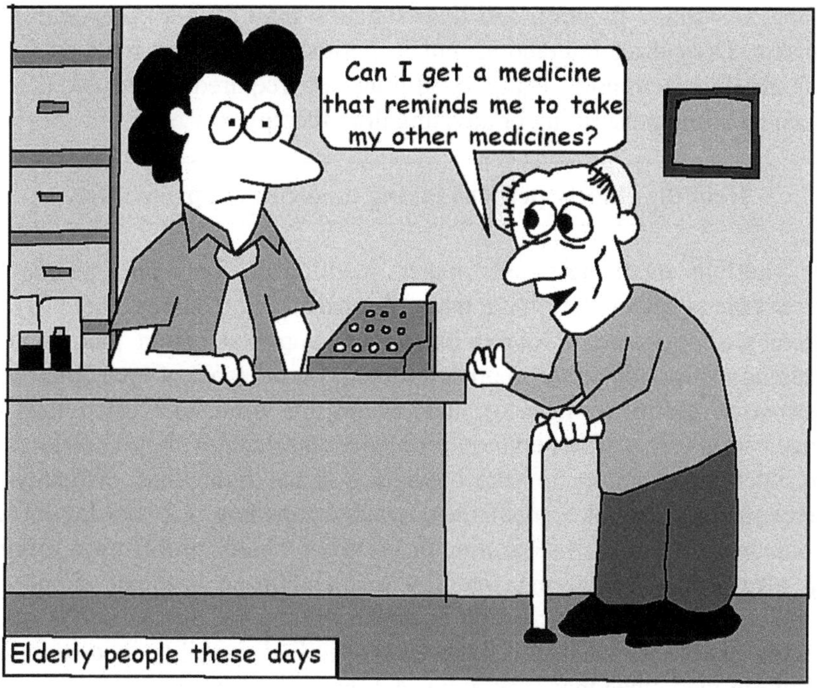
Can I get a medicine that reminds me to take my other medicines?
Elderly people these days

With improved economy together with increasing in accessibility of modern health care has increased the average life span of Indian population from 36.7 years in 1951 to 64.6 years in 2000. At present the elderly group (> 60 years) constitute around 7 % of the population. Multiple pathological conditions of this group made them to use several medicines together. At some or other point of time they may be using four or five prescription (even more) medicines together with couple of non-prescription medicines. It has been reported that up to 50 % of the older patients do not take medicines as intended.

With advancing age, there are physiologic and pathologic changes in human body. The decrease in body weight, decrease gastric secretion, change in body composition with reduced lean body mass and increased fat tissue, reduced renal flow etc., demands that the dosage regimen of many medicines be appropriately adjusted for elderly persons. The dose and/or frequency needs reduction in many cases failing which there would be overdosing with increasing side or adverse effects. The impaired kidney function and liver function may further complicate the matter. Drug-drug interaction and sometimes interaction with drinking (alcohol) is common. These conditions are required to be taken into account while prescribing or advising drug therapy.

Help the elderly persons taking medicines appropriately.

Multiple medicines' use makes it difficult for many people to remember whether they have taken the particular medicine. Inability to distinguish between coloured medicines, impaired vision that prevent reading instruction either in prescription or on the label of medicines, and decreased ability to hear or understands the directions often lead to medication errors. The common problems associated with medication use in elderly are: failure to take medicines at the right time, difficulty in remembering to take medicines, trouble opening the bottle, jar or container, difficulty in separating or breaking tablets, problems in mixing or measuring medications, inability to maintain an adequate supply of medicines, difficulty in reading or understanding the instruction or label, taking greater or smaller dosage than specified, inability to distinguish between medicines that look alike. All these can lead to unintentional in appropriate use of medicines. Not taking medicines or taking too little may confuse the doctor that the medicines are ineffective and he may change the drug therapy. On the other hand too much may cause adverse or toxic effects, even illness.

It is not that care is essential while taking prescription medicines only. There are several over the counter medicines, which may cause serious problems if not, used appropriately, especially in elderly population. An elderly person suffering from arthritis may be inclined to use analgesics or anti-inflammatory agents more frequently. Many of these medicines are associated with gastric bleeding which could be life threatening.

Antihistamines (anti-allergic) medicines dose sometimes get doubled if the patient is taking a cough and cold medicines containing antihistamine along with prescribed antihistamine. This can make the person dizzy or unsteady, leading to falls and broken bones. Antihistamines can sometimes cause confusion or delirium particularly in high doses or in combination with other medicines. Antacids containing aluminium are more likely to cause constipation and magnesium based antacids likely to cause diarrhoea.

While wise use of medicines can be beneficial for older people, number of factors contribute for their misuse and drug interaction leading to serous and undesirable side effects. As these group of patients require specialized drug treatment, and increasing number of such patients make the geriatric medicine practice (discipline) popular. The following simple tips are helpful for both the elderly patients and their family members in improving the medicines use:

- Elderly patient or family member must mention the OTC medicines to the doctor, the patient is using. The doctors will weigh the total drug regimen before prescribing.
- If you feel difficulty in following doctor's instruction, discuss the matter directly with him and do not act alone.
- Ask for details how to use medicines and insist for a written medication schedule or card.
- If you have swallowing problem, ask for liquid medicines.
- If the elderly person can not manage medicines properly, please keep the medicines away from them.

Approaching the problems of elderly with sensitivity and help by family members in medication use will help this group of population to lead more healthy life. It must be our duty too to help them in this stage of their life just as gratitude of their contributions, during most productive period, for making a better world for us.

CHAPTER 21

Medicines during Pregnancy (Are Medicines during Pregnancy Safe?)

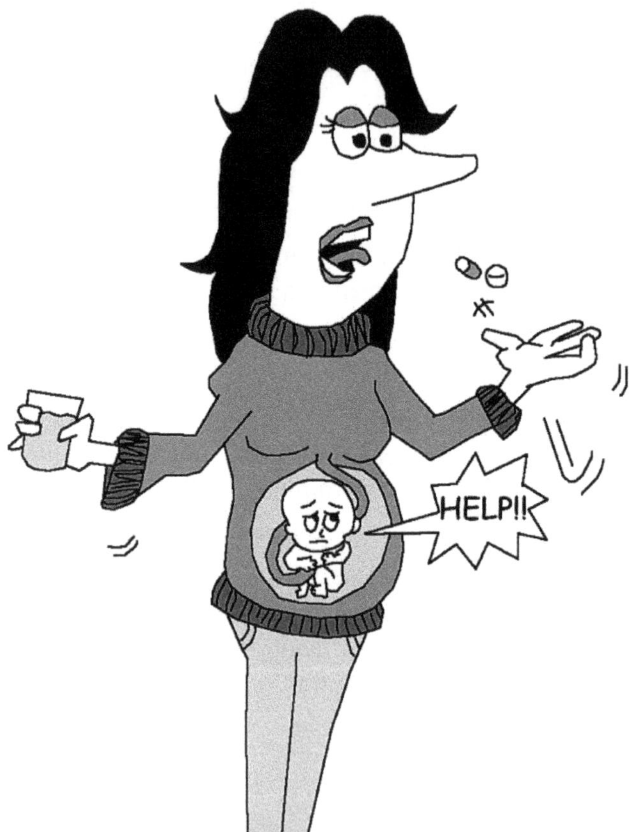

"Avoid self medication during pregnancy, Follow doctor's or pharmacist's Advice"

"Be careful about medicines, especially if you are pregnant, breast feeding or intending to become pregnant."

Women are special in our society and are usually responsible for caring for everyone in the family. Often they have disproportionately poor access to modern health care. Pregnancy is perhaps the most crucial and satisfying period in women's life. During this period the care of mother and the foetus is of utmost importance. As many medicines are known to cause adverse effects on mother and foetus, their use during this period requires careful evaluation of its effect on safety and efficacy on both.

Many medicines cross the placental barrier and reach fetus in the same way as the nutrients cross over from mother's blood to fetus blood. These medicines may affect the fetus in many ways: directly acting on the fetus causing damage, abnormal development and even death; altering the functions of placenta resulting in reduction in exchange of oxygen and nutrients between mother and foetus; or causing forceful contraction of uterus leading to injuring the foetus. The extent of such effects of medicine on fetus depends on development stage of foetus, potency of medicine and the dose.

The story of thalidomide disaster is well known in the history of medicine use in general and their use during pregnancy in particular. The birth defects resulted from thalidomide use in 1960s taught a painful lesson to the whole world that medicines should not be taken into granted that they all are safe and care must be exercised while using medicines during pregnancy.

Do not take any medicine during pregnancy and breast feeding without your doctor's advice.

The first trimester (three months from the day of conception) is the most vulnerable period and there is possibility of congenital malformation (teratogenesis). However during the second and third trimesters, medicines may affect the growth and functional development of the fetus or may have toxic effects on fetal tissues. Medicines administered or used shortly before the delivery too can affect on the labour or on the neonate after delivery.

Regulatory authorities (drugs control departments) of various countries have developed classification schemes for medicines based on their potential risk of possible teratogenic effects in various stages of pregnancy. There are no common schemes and unfortunately we do not have any such classification system in our country. The USA classification system divides medicines into five categories: A, B, C, D and X, based on their safety.

Categories	Comments
A	Adequate studies in pregnant women have not demonstrated a risk to fetus in the first trimester and there is no evidence of risk in later trimesters.
B	Animal studies have not demonstrated a risk to the fetus; there are no adequate studies in pregnant women. Or animal studies have shown adverse effects, but adequate studies on pregnant women have not demonstrated a risk to the fetus.
C	Animal studies have shown an adverse effect on the fetus but there are no adequate studies in humans. Benefits from the use of medicine may be acceptable despite the potential risk.
D	There is evidence of human fetal risk, but potential benefits from use of medicine in pregnant women may be acceptable despite its potential risk.
X	Studies in animals and humans demonstrate fetal abnormalities or fetal risk. The risk outweighs the potential benefits.

To sum off, the A categories of medicines are perhaps safe while the X categories are the most toxic to fetus. X categories are to be avoided during pregnancy. Alcohol, tetracyclines (antibiotics), coumarin (anticoagulants), Diethyl stilbosterol (DES) and lead are known teratogenics in humans.

Social drugs like nicotine in smoking and alcohol in drinks too have adverse effects on fetus. Low birth weight, miscarriage, stillbirths and premature births are common in among women who smoke during pregnancy. Drinking alcohol during pregnancy can cause birth defects.

Though during pregnancy mother and the foetus form a non-separable functional unit; maternal well being is absolute prerequisite in drug treatment. The treatment should aim at treating mother while protecting the foetus from the ill effects of the medicine. Though medicines can have harmful effects on foetus at any time during pregnancy, not using medicines out of fears may cause more harm. This may lead to not treating illness, maternal non-compliance with dosage schedule or course, sub optimal treatment and treatment failures.

Here are few tips:

- Tell your doctor, if you are pregnant or planning to be pregnant. Your doctor will prescribe accordingly.
- Avoid using medicines (including common ones) during pregnancy without doctor's advice.
- Avoid new medicines. Their safety is not well established.
- Prefer single component medicines.

Beside the risks involved, there are possibilities of changes in maternal medicine handling (the way body deals with medicine) during pregnancy because of multitude of physiological changes. Usually the doctor considers these changes while prescribing. The pregnant women should be informed of treatment choices and the accurate information would alleviate fears, improve patients' compliance leading to better treatment.

CHAPTER 22

Medicines during Breast Feeding (Avoid Medicines during Breast Feeding)

Breast-feeding is one of the oldest and healthiest practices of human civilization. It has been recommended that the infants be exclusively breast fed for at least first four months of life, and if possible, for six months. Mother's milk is the most ideal food. It not only provides the basic easily digestible and absorbable food, it also protects the baby from infection. Mother's defences against illness are passed onto the baby through her milk.

Most medicines pass into breast milk in very small and negligible amounts, so they do not harm the baby. In such case, it may be more harmful to stop breast-feeding while taking medicines. On the other hand many medicines taken by nursing mother pass into milk and even attain a much higher concentration than that of in maternal blood. Medicines may attain in much higher concentration, if nursing mother has decreased renal function (kidney problem). In these situations the baby is exposed to medicines' pharmacological and toxicological effects.

The medicines taken by nursing mother may affect the infant in many ways, if they pass in sufficient concentration: It may harm the infant (ergotamine – used in migraine), may inhibit lactation (estrogens – as contraceptive) causing less mother milk available for baby. Some medicines inhibit infant's sucking reflexes (Phenobarbital - used in epilepsy). The medicine in breast milk may cause hypersensitive reactions (allergy), even when the concentration is too low for producing pharmacological action. Tetracycline (antibiotic) excreted into milk may lead to deposition of the drug in bones and teeth causing discoloration of teeth.

Prolactin is a hormone that controls milk production and its level is increased after delivery. Infant feeding controls the serum prolactin level for adequate milk production. Medicines that decrease prolactin level in body cause a decrease in milk production affecting the baby's nutrition. Bromocriptine (used in parkinsonism), ergot alkaloids (used in migraine) and L-dopa (used in parkinsonism) belong to this category of medicines.

Do not take any medicine during pregnancy and breast feeding without your doctor's advice.

Whenever possible, nursing mothers should not take any medicine. Mothers who must take anti-thyroid medicines, lithium (used in mania), chloramphenicol (antibiotic), sulphonamides (antibacterial) and anticancer agents should not breast feed.

The extent to which the infant is at risk of adverse effects of medicines taken by nursing mother depends on the quantity of medicine excreted into the milk. The metabolic and excretory capacity (functions of liver and kidney) of the infant too plays important role. During drug development process through clinical trials, a drug is usually not administered to lactating woman. As a consequence, very little information on excretion of drug into human milk is available.

Though safety and efficacy (risk verses benefits) weighed carefully before using medicine during breast feeding, ultimate decision must be individualized based on illness and therapeutic options available. Few guidelines for safe and effective use of medicines during breast feeding:

- Ideally avoid using any medicine. If required, the medicines which are least excreted (or, excreted in minimum quantity) into milk should be of choice. Your doctor or pharmacist would have such knowledge.
- Action of medicines taken on chronic basis by mothers may be more harmful to infants than that of medicines taken for short time during acute illness.
- For long acting/sustained release medicines: Take medicines just prior to longest sleep period of the infant. When short acting forms of medicines are available, they should be preferred.
- Discontinue breast-feeding when contraindicated medicines are used.
- In your next visit tell your doctor that you are breast-feeding. Similarly tell your pharmacist while buying non-prescription medicines. They would select the safe one for you.

CHAPTER 23

Development of Medicines

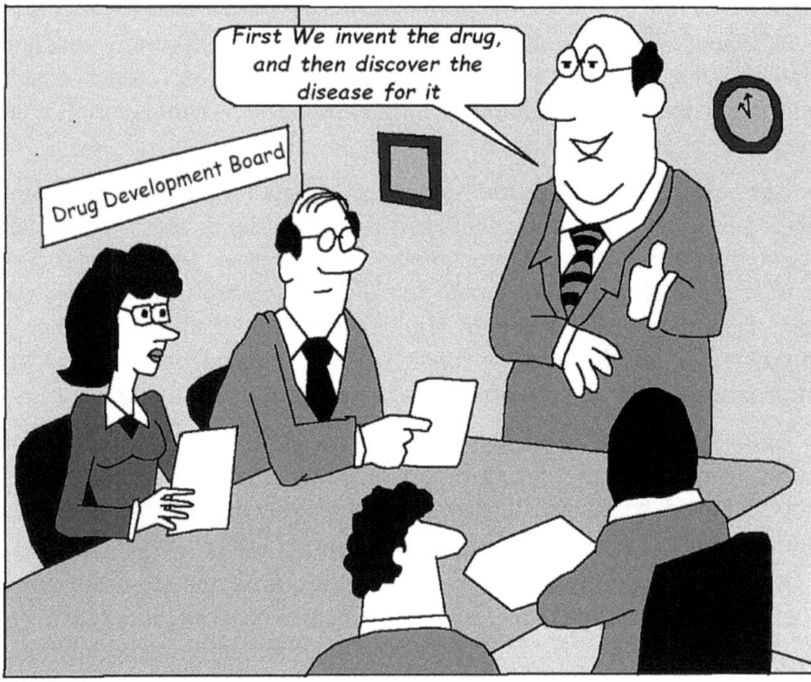
First We invent the drug, and then discover the disease for it
Drug Development Board

The role of medicines (or drugs) in saving lives, restoring health and preventing diseases or epidemics is well understood. In this article a brief process of developing medicine is discussed so that the consumers appreciate the need of appropriate use medicines they take or use.

New drugs are needed to fight the diseases for which no cure is available currently or as an alternative to existing drugs with improved safety and effectiveness, the two important requirements of drugs and drug therapy. Most of the new drugs are discovered by commercial pharmaceutical companies rather than in research or academic institutions. Drug discovery is a lengthy and tedious process, which takes about 5 to 10 years costing an average expenditure of $ 800 million.

Though many of the drugs in current use were discovered by experimental trial and observation in animals and human subjects, of late more rational approach is followed in drug discovery. Many of the drugs are obtained from herbal source, but synthetic organic compounds dominate the present drug market. Development in biotechnology and genetic engineering further improved the process of drug discovery.

Once a new compound shows promise, it is tested for its activity and safety. Initial study is carried out in several species of animals, called preclinical testing. Once the compound demonstrates the benefit is more than the risk involved in its use, it is ready for testing on human subjects called clinical trial. Permission is necessary for testing on human subjects. Permission is given normally on basis on animal testing report. The Drugs Controller General (India) is the authority to issue such permission in our country. Food and Drugs Administration is the equivalent body for USA.

The human testing is conducted in three phases: Phase – I, Phase – II and Phase – III under the supervision of medically qualified scientists or professionals. Phase – I is testing of new compound in limited number of healthy volunteers to assess safety and dosage. On an average only 5 out of 250 compounds crosses this barrier. Once the safety and dosage is established, phase – II study can begin. It is carried out in limited number of patients to evaluate effectiveness and to look for side effects. The phase –III is conducted in large number of patients in several centers to verify effectiveness and monitor adverse reactions from long-term use. Only 1 in 5 compounds tested pass this phase to get into the market for use. On scrutinization of the clinical trial data the approvals for the compound is given for marketing.

Though many of the medicines available today are discovered after experimental trials, of late more rational approach is followed in drug discovery.

Though the drug reaches the market after a careful and thorough screening, many of the side effects or toxic effects are not noticed during these three phases of study. It is essential to continue monitoring the drug for detecting possible toxic response of drug on long-term use, called post marketing surveillance. A classical example of benefit of such study is withdrawal of rofecoxib, a painkiller from USA market and later banning the use of it in our country.

The development process continues for optimizing the drug delivery through various routes. The consumers need to be vigilant while they use drugs, whether old or new, and report back the experienced side effects to the doctors and pharmacovigilance centres established recently under Central Drugs Control Organization. They too require to use medicines wisely as lot of resources are spent developing them.

CHAPTER 24

Clinical Trials

New medicines are needed to fight the diseases for which no cure is available at present, or as an alternative to existing medicines with improved safety and effectiveness. The development of new medicines is a lengthy, risky and tedious process. The experimental medicinal substance can't be directly tested on human beings. The animal testing data (pre-clinical testing) forms the foundation for the clinical testing. The testing of experimental medicinal substance passed through the preclinical phase is a potential candidate for testing on human beings. The animal models can not completely simulate the disease conditions of human beings and the experimental toxicity data obtained from animals can't be extrapolated either to humans. Hence testing of promising medicinal substance in humans is a must before being approved for mass use as medicine. The testing of this new substance in healthy human beings and then on patients is known as clinical trial.

The clinical trial has three distinct phases which must be carried out before the test medicinal substance is approved for mass use. The clinical trial cannot be carried out without the permission of the Drugs Controller General India. The Drugs Controller General is the Head of the Central Drugs Standard Control Organization, the Department responsible for maintaining the quality and standards of medicines in this country. In addition to this permission, the approval from ethics committee is also essential to carry out clinical trials. Out of three phases mentioned above, the phase – I is performed in healthy human volunteers. While the other two phases: phase II and phase – III are carried out in patients.

Clinical Trials are human experimentations in drug discovery. Understand the risks and benefits before giving consent to participate in clinical trials.

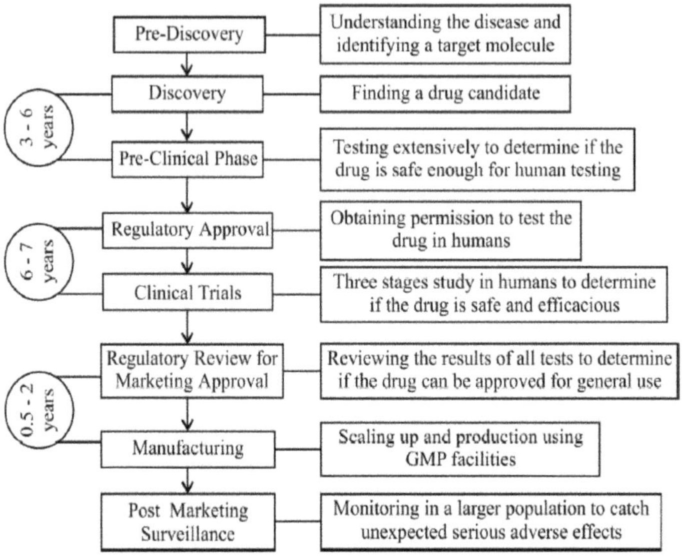

The phase – I study is initial human testing in a small group of healthy human beings, termed as volunteers. The number of healthy volunteers participate in the study vary from 20 to 100. The study aimed at deciding the safe dosing range which can be used for next phase study. For the first time, the effects of the substance as well as how body handles it are studied in humans.

The phase –II is a controlled clinical study in a small group of patients ranging from 100 to 500 in number with disease to assess the test medicinal substance's effectiveness, side effects and risks. Each patient is monitored as dose is increased. This phase of study aims to decide what is the minimum dose required to produce a beneficial effect and what is the maximum dose that produce severe undesirable effects.

The phase – III is a controlled and uncontrolled clinical trial involving around 1000 – 5000 patients to generate statistically data about safety, efficacy and overall benefit – risk relationship of the test medicinal substances. The results of the study are the basis for approval of the test substance as medicine for mass use.

Based on animal testing, the Drugs Controller General of India allows the initiation of clinical trials. The permission for clinical trials is issued successively based on the outcome of the previous phase. Finally, after the phase – III study demonstrates that the use of substance has more beneficial effects than the risks involved in using it, permission is granted to market the medicine. However, the study does not end here. The clinical trials are limited study and many of the adverse effects of medicines cannot be captured. When the medicines are used in large scale after marketing permission, often many adverse effects are noticed. If serious side effects appear, the decision is often taken to restrict its use or ban its use (withdrawing the medicine from the market). This phase of study that is continued after marketing approval is called phase – IV study or Post-Marketing Surveillance. The post marketing surveillance is meant for monitoring adverse effects of medicines during use.

While the clinical trials are useful to protect the people from large scale exposure from unsafe medicines, the people who participate in these studies need to be treated with dignity and protected from exploitation. Hence, the Government of India outlines the Ethical Guidelines to be followed in carrying out biomedical experiments on human beings including clinical trials. The basic principles of the ethical guideline are to safe guard the interest of human subjects participating in clinical trials. These four basic principles are: *Beneficence* (this requires that good should result, harm should be avoided, or that the benefits should justify the risk or harm, *Non-Maleficence* (do no harm), *Respect for rights* (this requires that the human subjects have free choice whether to participate or not), and *Justice* (this requires an equal distribution of burden and benefit). These basic principles of ethics are universal and followed throughout the world.

India is being increasingly seen as sites for clinical trials. A large number of trials are now ongoing mostly global ones. The people of India are often alleged to have been treated as experimental guinea pigs even if the strict regulations are in force. The ethical guidelines are reported to have violated and the trials are conducted without the permission of the Drugs Controller. These are the cases of our ignorance leading to exploitation. The general understanding of clinical trials not only help us while carrying out clinical trials in scientific and ethical way but also protect us from being exploited while participating is such research as participants.

CHAPTER 25

Be Informed before Participating in Clinical Trials

It has been recently reported that more than 1100 people died during clinical trials in 2010 and 2011. Many of these deaths are attributed to the serious adverse events though few were only compensated. This caused a lot of concern both within and outside the parliament. In order to appropriately compensate the person affected or harmed during clinical trials, the Government of India has just issued draft guidelines for calculating the extent of compensation.

India now becomes the favourite destination for international clinical trials. The estimated size of the Indian clinical trial market was $ 250-300 million during 2010. Lower cost, a huge population "treatment naïve", large pool of trained health professionals and numerous world-class medical facilities are in favour of India. Several contract research organisations (CRO) are being established for conducting drug research in human beings. There are often reports that the Indian patients are treated like guinea pigs and illegal studies are common.

It is possible that many healthy individuals as well as patients would participate (or, may be already participating) in the clinical trials as volunteers. The CROs would be recruiting volunteers for the drug testing. The individuals need to know the risks involved, if participated, and their rights while participating as volunteers. A knowledgeable and well-informed individual can take decision whether to participate or not, while innocent and ignorant people are likely to fall into this trap.

An understanding of the clinical trial process would help the prospective volunteers to take informed decision and participate in a responsible way. Clinical trial is the study of new drug in human in order to assess its safety and efficacy. The clinical trials can only be conducted after permission from the Drugs Controller General, India, and ethics committee of the institution. If the animal testing confirmed the benefits of drugs compared to risks associated, then only the experiments in human beings are allowed. The detail guidelines to be followed are outlined in schedule Y (recently amended) of Drugs and Cosmetics Act, 1940. The study conducting authority must comply with Good Practices in clinical research as specified by government of India. Good Clinical (Research) Practice (GCP) aims at conducting international quality research for generating valid and reliable safety and efficacy data while offering public assurance of protecting the rights, safety and well being of the participating subjects.

The study is conducted at three stages: phase – I (only on healthy volunteers), phase – II (on limited number of patients) and phase - III (in large number of patients at different centres). The permission to continue too is accorded on stages. The study is designed in such a way that the patient may either get the new drug under testing, a standard drug or a dummy drug.

Besides knowing the risk and benefits, you should know whom to contact in emergency if you plan to participate in clinical trial.

The institutional ethics committee, before commencement of the trial, usually approves the study protocol and design. The ethics committee consists of several members in whom at least there would be representation from legal expertise, social science and general lay public. It is the responsibility of the investigators to inform the ethics committee of any serious adverse effect(s) of the experimental drug noticed or experienced by the participating subjects. The individuals are required to sign the ethics committee approved informed consent form. These forms must be made available to the intending volunteers in their understandable languages, preferably in mother tongue indicating the details of the study like purpose, protocol, duration, number of people participating, evaluation process, benefits and compensation. The intending persons should know the alternate treatment procedure available, the risks involved and likely benefits for participating. "What compensation and/or treatment available in the event of trial related injury; the anticipated prorated money, anticipated expenses?" should be the important concern of the individual.

The informed consent form is either signed by the prospective volunteer himself or herself or by the legal guardian. The particulars of subjects and data are required to be kept confidential unless asked under court of law.

More than 140 medicinal products have been withdrawn from various markets around the globe over last four decades because of actual or perceived safety cause. The most frequent problems are reported to be associated with liver, blood and heart disorders.

While clinical trials are justified for developing newer, safer and better drugs for the future, the participating subjects should be regarded as full partners by keeping them well informed. This would place them in better position to make decisions whether to participate or not and continuation in the study.

Before participating or enrolling, you must know the following (ask the doctor concerned):

- What risk is involved either in participating volunteer/embryo/fetus/or nursing infant?
- Confirm about the compensation provision available in case of adverse or serious adverse events.
- What are expected benefits of the study?
- Remember the name of investigator (doctor) and emergency contact number.
- Thoroughly read and understand the consent form. If required do not hesitate to ask the form in your mother tongue.
- You can leave the study at any point of time without assigning any reason. This would not affect your regular treatment or legal rights. Check this before signing the consent form.
- Inform your unusual experience immediately to the investigator (doctor).

Compensation in case of trial related injury or death:

- In case of injury, the trail participants are entitled for free medical management as long as required.
- Participants are also entitled for financial compensation over and above any expenses incurred on medical management.
- Financial compensation is to be paid to the nominee of the participants, in case of death.
- The Drugs Controller General of India decides the quantum of financial compensation.
- The compensation varies from a minimum of Rs 2 Lakh to maximum of Rs 73.60 Lakh.

CHAPTER 26

New Drugs: Pros and Cons

A few weeks ago, one of doctor friends' wife was narrating the sufferings they underwent for buying a latest technology driven refrigerator. They purchased the piece just four years back at a premium price and now when they need a service, the company is found to be no more in the business. This made them to buy again a new refrigerator after disposing the old one at a throwaway price. This is a good lesson for every consumer and is more relevant to medicine.

The new drugs are the medicines, which are recently introduced for use. Legally they are treated as new drugs till the four years from the date of approval for use. Their safety is not well established. Every medicine carries with it some degree of benefits for which medicine is useful on one hand and risk on the other. Sometimes the risk outweighs the benefits. None is entirely safe.

The medicines are tested, in a limited extent, both in animals and human beings for efficacy and safety before getting approved for general use. But such study does not tell the whole truth. We find this recently when a painkiller "rofecoxib" is banned in our country. The drug was first withdrawn by the inventing company from USA market as it was found to have serious heart related problems including death.

New drugs are to be used with caution and are preferred only when the alternatives are ineffective or not available.

The patients and healthy human beings are sometimes recruited as volunteers for testing of new drugs (pre marketing). They must be extra careful before consenting to take part in this type of study. At a minimum, they need to know the risk involved and the compensation amount in case unfortunate severe events happen. Even when the new drugs are prescribed, the consumers must exercise their rights asking for alternatives. They are required only when the time tested and long standing drugs are found to be ineffective. They are normally aggressively promoted and the people fall into the trap as they have fancy for new things.

New medicines are not tested on children or pregnant women before approval. These categories of patients need to extra careful. The world has experienced the use of thalidomide (a sleeping tablet of 1960) in pregnant women resulting in birth deformities in babies. Soon after, the drug was withdrawn. These are not the only drugs but there are many, which are withdrawn from market following detection of severe risks associated with their use.

Testing in animals and limited trial on human beings are insufficient to predict complete human safety. One needs to remember that medicine is to be used when necessary and has to be careful as it can harm or even kill.

CHAPTER 27

Drink and Medicines

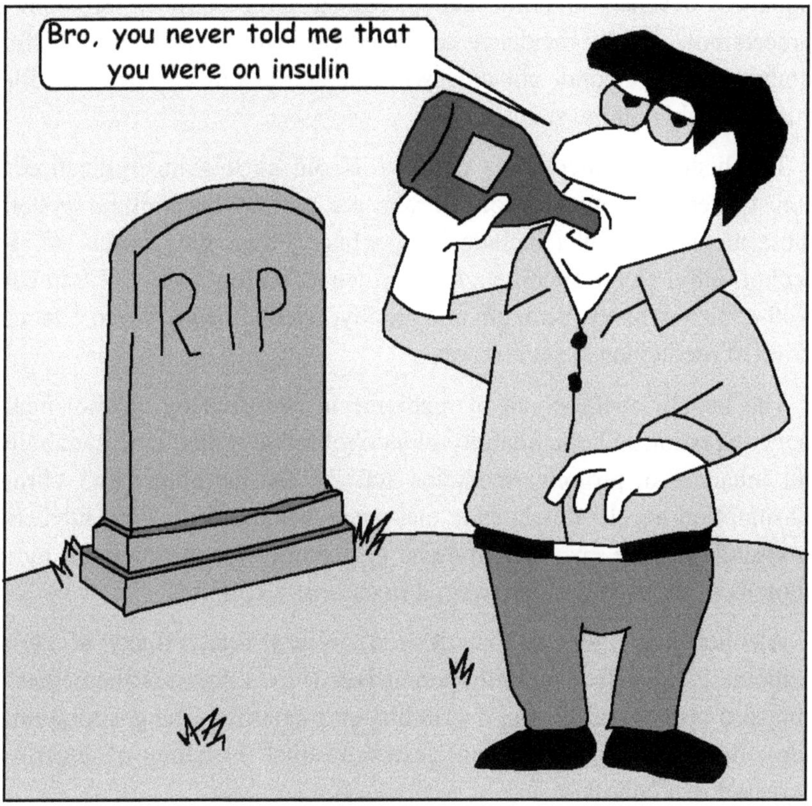
Bro, you never told me that you were on insulin
RIP

"Never take alcohol when on insulin"

(a) On Medication - Then keep off Alcohol)

A heavy drinker is hospitalized after using paracetamol tablets for treating his backache. The reason is liver toxicity. Why did it happen? It happened because alcohol had increased liver toxicity problem of paracetamol. High incidence of medical emergencies arises from combination of alcohol not only with medicines but also with all illicit drugs available on the street.

The history of alcohol is perhaps as old as human civilization. In almost every society alcoholic drinks are part of the cultural systems. These alcoholic drinks include beer, whisky, rum, gin, arrack etc. The alcohol (ethyl alcohol) content of them varies widely from 5-7% in beers to 40-45% in whisky, rum, gin and brandy. Alcohol is known to affect the action of medicines in several ways.

The hepatic metabolism of medicine is modified by alcohol intake. Acute ingestion of large quantity of alcohol reduces medicine metabolism and enhances or prolongs medicine activity. On the other hand, chronic consumption accelerates hepatic clearance (removal) of some medicines by stimulating the enzymes systems responsible for metabolism. Larger amounts of these drugs are required in chronic alcoholics.

Alcohol may enhance the desired or undesired effects of certain medicines. The effect of antihypertensives (blood pressure medicines) is increased because of alcohol's vasodilation properties. The gastrointestinal side effects like gastritis and gastrointestinal bleeding of aspirin is increased in alcoholics.

Alcohol influences the action of many medicines and even potentiates their toxicity.

The alcohol affects the action of medicines by some other methods too. Here is just a small list of alcohol and medicine interaction:

Medicine	Used for	Effect of Interaction
Paracetamol	Pain and fever	Increased risk of liver damage
Antihistamines	Cold, allergy etc.	Excessive sedation that could be fatal
Phenytoin	Epilepsy	Reduced drug effectiveness
Insulin	Diabetes	Excessive low blood sugar
Penicillin	Bacterial infection	Reduced therapeutic effectiveness
Diazepam	Minor tranquilizer, sedative	Potentiates clinical effects
Aspirin	Pain, fever and inflammation	Potentiates the risk of gastric irritation and bleeding
Promethazine	Vomiting	Potentiates central nervous system depression
INH	Tuberculosis	Risk of hepatitis is high especially over 50 years
Metronidazole	Bacterial and protozoal infection	Nausea, vomiting, headache etc.

In short, the alcohol either increases or decreases medicine activity and may increases the undesirable or toxic effects of medicines. There are many medicines that are affected by alcohol ingestion. One has to be especially careful while taking sleeping medications, antianxiety, antidepressants, antihistamines, certain blood pressure medications, antiarthritic, blood thinners and antidiabetic medicines. Thus it is dangerous to drink alcohol while taking certain medicines.

It is not that alcohol affects the medicine activity. The reverse is also true. Medicines can influence alcohol breakdown by altering levels of enzyme, alcoholdehydrogenase. Aspirin when taken on full stomach reduces enzyme level by one half, causing more alcohol to accumulate in the blood. Such effect is more in women than men. Gastric ulcer medications also inhibit this enzyme and increase the physiological effect of alcohol.

Beside the direct actions of alcohol on medicines, there are other problems too. During drinking bouts and blackout spells, patients sometimes forget to take their medications or take more than the prescribed amount. Former leads to poor patients' compliance with no or reduced drug action while the latter may lead to overdosing.

With widespread use of alcohol in general population, doctors and the pharmacists must always keep ethanol – drug interaction in mind while advising patients. The patients should also behave in a responsible manner and tell the doctor or pharmacist about his habit of drinking. This is in best interest of patients. If possible avoid drinking while on therapy. Or else, at least enquire about possible interaction of medicines you are taking and alcohol.

(b) Medication with Drink Endangers Health!

Kahani me Twist. “The death of wife of a high profile political leader was accidental and self-induced and caused by the prolonged intake of acetaminophen while consuming alcohol” an eminent forensic scientist said. The case is still under investigation and cause of death is yet to be confirmed. But this is true! The combination of acetaminophen (also called paracetamol) and alcoholic drinks endangers your health.

Paracetamol is one of the most common household medicines. This is used for relieving fever and pain. But the medicine is very toxic too. You may be surprised to know “the paracetamol is used to induce liver toxicity in experimental animals”. More than 4 gram per day which means eight tablets of 500 mg strength is not advisable as it may lead to serious liver problems. Alcohol further increases this liver toxicity. United States Food and Drugs administration warns “If you consume 3 or more alcoholic drinks every day, you should ask your doctor whether you should take acetaminophen (paracetamol) or other pain relievers/fever reducers”. While the paracetamol itself is not that toxic but its metabolite is more problematic. Alcohol induces the metabolic enzyme and thereby increases the liver toxicity of paracetamol.

The history of alcohol use is perhaps as old as human civilization. This has perhaps started with Soma Rasa. The modern alcoholic drinks include beer, whisky, rum, gin, arrack etc. The alcohol (ethyl alcohol) content of them varies widely from 5-7 % in beers to 40-45 5% in whisky, rum, gin and brandy. There has been disturbing trend in the growth of alcoholic drinks. The recent World Health Organization reported “An average Indian male drinker takes around 33 litres of alcohol a year while the average women drinker consumes 11 litres”. This statistics of 2012 is higher than that of 2008. The alcohol consumption is much higher than even the developed countries where people regularly drink and drinking in society ia acceptable. Americans consume 8.5 to 9.9 liters of alcohol per annum while the Canadians consume 12.5 liters per annum. Alcohol is responsible for many human hazards. It is known to be the cause of 60 different types of diseases.

Alcohol is known to affect the action of many medicines in several ways. Aspirin and Ibuprofen, the two common pain killers, too are contraindicated in heavy drinkers. Both are harmful to gastric mucosa and they damage causing ulceration. Narcotic analgesics too are incompatible combination with alcohol as there are possibilities of respiratory depression. The sedatives have additive effects in combination with alcohol. Alcohol increases the health hazards of persons taking illegal recreational drugs. The list often is endless. On the other hand, medicines adversely affect the activity of alcohol. Metronidazole, a medicine for amoebiasis and treating some bacterial infection, causes disulfiram-like reactions, a very unpleasant experience for drinkers.

Many Ayurvedic medicine preparations contain high quantity of alcohol. These preparations too equally risky like drinks. It is not just that the drink influences the action of medicines. The reverse is also equally true. While it may be difficult to know which medicine have potential interaction problem without your doctor's/pharmacist's advice, it is preferable to take a healthy decision to keep off alcoholic drinks while on medication.

CHAPTER 28

Food and Medicines (Does Food affect Medicine?)

One of the readers of my column has asked me why are some medicines are to be taken in empty stomach while many are advised to be taken after food or meal. This article is in response to this query and how do our diets influence medicines' activity is the content of this article.

The importance of food in daily life needs no emphasis. In the global campaign for Health for All, nutrition is one of the eight elements of primary health care. While a balance diet containing a variety of foods in adequate quantity and proportion met the nutritional requirements of healthy life and prevent dietary deficiency diseases, some of the food that we eat may make some medicines work faster or slower or even prevent them from having any effect.

Foods affect the medicines at different stages of medicines' journey in the body. When we swallow medicine, the food present in the stomach influences its entry into the blood, a process medically known as absorption. The medicine needs to be absorbed adequately and appropriate rate to produce clinical effect. For some medicines, there is no influence of food on absorption, while absorption of many medicines is greatly influenced. The presence of food causes a reduction of absorption of antiinfective medicine, amoxicillin. Calcium containing food such as milk, cheese and other dairy products reduces the extent of absorption of tetracyclines, antibacterial medicine. The clinical effects of both the medicines are reduced. Absorption of most of the medicines is better and more predictable when taken in empty stomach and with large volume of water. However, Griseofulvin, an antifungal antibiotic, is better absorbed if taken after a fatty meal. There are another group of medicines like iron salts, non steroidal anti-inflammatory medicines (pain killers); are required to be taken always after food in order to reduce the undesirable gastric irritation effects of these medicines. Timing of medicines is very essential in order to avoid the effects of food on medicines action. When medicines are advised to be taken before food, they should be taken at least one hour before or two hours after eating.

Before food means: Take medicines 30 minutes before taking food or take after 2 hours of taking food.

Food is also reported to affect the clearance (elimination from the body) of theophylline, an asthma medicine. Dietary in takeoff charcoal broiled food (beef) and high protein diets are associated with increased theophylline elimination, while high carbohydrate diets decrease elimination. Increased or decreased clearance may require dosage adjustment. The diet rich in vitamin K (couli flower, beans, spinach, pork, fish etc.) may antagonize the effects of warfarin (anticoagulant) requiring dose adjustment of warfarin.

It is not that we need to avoid certain foods during drug therapy. It is also important to take certain foods while on drug therapy. Diuretics like furosemide have tendency to deplete potassium from body. Potassium is an important mineral needed for proper body function. In such situation, it is advisable to take potassium rich diet like dried apricots, bananas, dates, beans, potatoes, soybeans etc., to restore excess potassium lost, unless one is on potassium supplement. Of course, there are diuretics, which have no potassium depletion affect.

Here is a list of some potentially harmful food-medicine interactions:

Medicine	Food	Interaction effect
Tetracycline (antibiotic)	Calcium containing: milk, cheese, yogurt; Iron rich: meat, beef liver, nuts, lettuce, spinach etc.	Effectiveness is interfered
Warfarin (prevent blood clotting)	Vitamin K containing: Liver and spinach	Effectiveness is interfered
Monoamine oxidase (MAO) inhibitors (to counter depression and high blood pressure)	Tyramine containing: aged cheese, chicken livers, fermented sausages, yogurt, beef liver etc.	Blood Pressure increased to dangerous level
Nefedipine (blood pressure medicine)	Grape Juice	Effect of drug is high leading to more lowering of blood pressure
Diazepam, lorazepam (tranquilizer, sedative)	Grape Juice	Increased sedative effects

In order to avoid the undesirable affect of food on medicines, follow your doctor's advice regarding when to take medicine: with food, after food, or before food; and what foods are to be avoided or what food should be taken. Do always report to your doctor about unusual experience or complaints that occur when you consume certain foods, while on drug therapy.

CHAPTER 29

Home Medicines Kit

With information explosion both in print and electronic media and increased cost of visiting doctor made many people more responsible than ever before for maintenance of their health. They are developing the expertise to prevent or manage numerous types of illness, injuries and conditions. Such knowledge and expertise are really essential and life saving when some health problem develops in the middle of night with no doctors nearby or it may be difficult to reach for medical facility in these odd hours. A medical emergency may even arise when natural disaster strikes. In all such situations, medicines available at your home, the home medicine kit, comes to your rescue.

There is nothing like ideal inventory for home medicine kit. It varies and depends on the nature, size, life style, location, age and health status of the individual and family. Having key medicines available and knowing how to use them will prevent delays in treating discomforting symptoms. These items may prevent costly and unnecessary trip to the doctor's clinic or casualty of the hospital, and avoid inconvenience; but they are not substitutes for proper medical attention.

In addition to the essential medicines, the kit should contain some first aid materials too. These items are required to manage cuts, scrapes, bites, stings, sprains and strains. The medicines include remedy for cold and allergy; gastrointestinal disturbances; pain and fever and common eye and ear problems. Antihistamines (chlorphenarmine maleate) and decongestants (pseudoephedrine) provide symptomatic relief to allergic rhinitis and common colds. Antihistamines treat allergic problems too. Heartburn and acid indigestion may be relieved by use of gastric antacids. Oral Rehydration Salts prevent dehydration and maintain electrolyte balance in diarrhoea. Antiemetics (domperidone) prevent vomiting. Antispasmodics (dicyclomine) can treat spasms in gastrointestinal tract (Pain in abdomen). Fever and pain including toothache can be treated with paracetamol and aspirin. Aspirin is not to be given to children. In a suspected heart attack, an aspirin tablet can be given before shifting to hospital. Eye drop may belong to antibacterial (ciprofloxacin). Ear pain can be treated with anti-inflammatory ear drop. Antibacterial and antinflammatory common drop for both eye and ear use is available and is preferred than separate eye drop and ear drop.

Periodically monitor the kit to detect expired medicines and replace them with fresh ones.

Kit Inventory

First aid items	Medicines*
A bandage roll A roll of cotton Few band aids Pain reliving ointment/spray Povidone iodine ointment Liquid antiseptic Thermometer Blunt scissor	Chlorphenarmine maleate tablets (antihistamine) Diphenhydramine tablets (decongestants)(may be in combination) Domperidone tablets (for vomiting) Antacid tablets (for heart burn and acidity) ORS packets (to prevent dehydration and maintain electrolyte balance) Dicyclomine tablets (for gastrointestinal spasm) Paracetamol tablets (for fever and pain) Aspirin tablets (for fever and pain) Antibacterial and anti-inflammatory eye/ear drop

* (Quantity should be either one strip or at least for two days requirement. Liquid preparations are essential for children.)

Important Tips for safe management of the kit

- Be familiar with the use of each item in the kit. Knowledge on dose and method of administration or use is essential. You can check these with your doctor or pharmacist.
- Keep the kit in an easily accessible place but out of reach of children.
- Keep it in a cool and dry place as temperature and humidity may accelerate the deterioration of medicines. Never keep in kitchen or bathroom.
- Periodically check the kit and remove or discard old, expired items and replace them with new stocks.
- Throw away the items that have changed colour, consistency or odour. Probably they become unfit for use or spoiled.
- If symptoms do not respond to treatment or worsen rapidly after being treated, do not hesitate to contact or consult your doctor.

CHAPTER 30

Medicines during Travel (For Safe Travel, Pack Your Medicines Too!)

Tourism today is one of the world's fasted growing industries. Aggressive tourism marketing, liberalized economy ties with better bilateral relationship have increased the people's mobility. Millions travel worldwide and many do within the country. While traveling is a pleasure, if together with family and friends, but often causes lot of inconvenience for sudden illness. As travel is properly planned to carry all necessary items, it is also similarly necessary to carry necessary and essential medicines to take care of sudden illness. Carrying of medicines is essential because similar medicines may not be available at destination place, or may be available in other name, which is often not known to the general public, the medicines often are sold only on the prescription of medical practitioners, or they may be required even during travel.

What medicines are to be carried is always a question. There is no universal list. Of course, two main factors influence the selection: the prevalence of disease condition of destination place and the individual's or family's health needs. Going to malaria prone area necessitates the carrying of anti-malarial medicines. People suffering from chronic conditions like asthma, diabetes etc. needs to carry their medicines. The most common problems people face is gastrointestinal infections resulting from contaminated drinking water, beverages, eating uncooked or undercooked food. The casual sexual contact can produce a high risk of infection with HIV. The following medicines are recommended to be kept in the medicines' kit (though not exhaustive): Analgesics (pain killers); Gastric antacids; anti-diarrhoeals and ORS; preventive care items such as insect repellant, anti-malarial drugs, sunscreen and condoms; antibiotics; first aid items like antiseptics, dressings and band aids; and medicines already taking for chronic conditions.

Carry the necessary medicines and the prescription while travelling to avoid inconvenience.

The travelers should transport their medicines in the original containers with intact labels wherever feasible. They should be carried in both hand baggage and luggage. Ideally the hand baggage should have sufficient medicines to cover the length of travel period. The storage of medicines during travel is another important consideration. Temperature adversely affects some medicines and they are required to be kept in refrigerator. Thyroxine, though advised to be stored in refrigerator at 2 to 8 °C, they are stable at below 25 °C for around 4 weeks. There is no need of panic. But the medicines must be used within 4 weeks only and after that they should be discarded. Insulin is also stable for several months at room temperature.

Buying medicines in overseas is often problem. There may be confusion on brand names. As brand names vary from country to country, the traveler needs to know the generic name of the medicines. The medicines are perhaps the cheapest in our country and their cost is several folds in developed countries. Even they are costlier in neighboring countries. The rules and regulations relating to medicines are very strict in certain countries. The medicines cannot be purchased like in India. Here almost every medicine is available across the counter. Certain medicines have legal problems. The medicines containing codeine (present in some cough preparations) are illegal in United Arab Emirates.

Here are few practical tips for carrying medicines during travel:

- Ensure that you have sufficient quantity of medicines for the entire length of travel: adequate quantities for your chronic condition and unexpected illness.
- Learn the proper use of medicines: dose and duration.
- Make sure that the medicines do not expire during travel.
- Transport them in original container and labels. It would help the custom to clear materials easily.
- Be familiar with legal restriction of certain medicines in the country of visit.
- Ideally divide your medicines into hand luggage and checked luggage. The hand luggage should have sufficient quantity to cover duration of travel and several days afterwards in case of delayed arrival of checked luggage.
- Carry a doctor's prescription indicating your requirement.

CHAPTER 31

Combination Medicines (Fixed Dose Combination Medicines – How useful they are!)

"Each tablet contains nimesulide –100 mg, pseudoephiedrine hydrochloride –120 mg, cetirizine – 5 mg". "Each 5 ml of the preparation contains chlorpheniramine maleate 1.25 mg, pseudoephedrin – 15 mg, paracetamol - 125 mg, guaiphenesin – 50 mg". These are the labels of medicinal products informing what medicinal constituents it has. Often we find the medicines contain more than one medicinally active ingredient. A product containing two or more active ingredients in a fixed proportion is called a fixed dose combination (FDC) product. Two or more medicinal ingredients combined in the same tablet or capsule or liquid preparation.

When two or more drugs are combined in a product they may interact with each other. Two drugs in combination may produce an effect that is greater than the effect of either drug administered alone. The combination effect may be just additive. In some cases the combined effect is more than summation of individual effect, hyper additive. These types of effects are medically called synergism and they are beneficial. There are increased risks of toxicity too with combination medicines.

The FDC medicinal products offer both advantages and as well as disadvantages. They are useful if there is medical rationale for combinations. The combination has a greater efficacy than any of the individual components given alone in same dose. For antimicrobials, the combinations results in reduced chances of resistance. FDC medicinal products (also as kit, not as exact sense FDC) are recommended for Tuberculosis, malaria and HIV (AIDS). The FDCs offer convenience for prescribers and patients. The patients will have less number of tablets (or, similar medicines) to be swallowed. This promotes better patients adherence to drug therapy, an important component in successful therapy. The improved adherence also reduces the chance of developing resistance especially with antimicrobials. The resistance threat is a global public health problem. These medicines cost less than the summation cost of individual component products. They offer simplified logistics of medicine procurement and distribution in public health system.

On the other hand, the fixed dose combination medicines have potential disadvantages too. The patients may be taking unnecessarily combination products while actually requiring only one or so. There is possibility of higher incidence or greater severity of adverse reactions to the combinations than individual ingredients given alone. Dose adjustment may be a problem as it is to be done for all components. The products are often unusually large and are difficult to swallow.

Though rational fixed drug combinations are useful and becoming increasingly important in the management of HIV/AIDS, malaria and tuberculosis, the combination offers improved patients' adherence to the treatment plan and reduced chances of developing resistance for antimicrobial agents. But irrational combination medicines are threat to public health. They impose unnecessary financial burden and often cause decreased quality of life. The Indian medicinal market is flooded with irrational combination medicines. Over the years many have been withdrawn. Nutritional supplements, cough and cold medicines, dermatological products, vitamins are most common groups of combination medicines. Anti-bacterials (gatifloxacin) with ornidazole for treatment of diarrhoea and dysentery of mixed origin, anti-bacterials with lactobacillus, paracetamol with antihistamines, gastric antacids with medicines to prevent stomach cramps, cough syrups containing both cough suppressants and expectorants, are just few examples of objectionable combinations. There are plenty.

Many of the Fixed Dose Combinations available in Indian Market have no rationality. Rational FDCs should only be used.

The use of medicines is often sentimental. In a casual discussion with some of my students reveal that many even prefer combination paracetamol products for just relieving fever. Paracetamol with cetirizine was the choice for one. It is not that the fever is always associated with running nose or cold. Why does one need both paracetamol and cetirizine? This is common in self-medication. Like buying one and taking one free. The mindset needs to be changed. The medicines are to be taken or used if only required and unnecessary use may cause harmful effects.

Legally speaking a new FDC is treated as new drug and requires evaluation of safety and efficacy as a combination product. The poor implementation of our regulation is responsible for irrational and unsafe medicines in the market. But the consumers need to be careful. Please remember:

- While buying medicines check the generic name. Brand name often would be confusing.
- Insist on single ingredient medicines rather than combination medicines, unless required. As an empowered consumer, it is essential to ask the doctor of the rationality of combination medicines if prescribed. May be it is difficult.
- They are expensive.
- The unnecessary components that you do need are burden to your system. The vital organs like liver and kidneys have to work hard for their removal.

CHAPTER 32

Advertisement on Medicines (Say No to AD Treatment)

One of the readers of my column "Know Your Medicine" has conveyed his sufferings after taking medicines based on advertisements for a cure for piles. He is not the lone personality having such an experience; many others too might have similar experience or no remedy at all. In this article I would like to alert the readers on dangerous aspects of medicine advertisement. The public should not become victims or prey to such advertisements.

In this electronic age, advertisements are part and parcel of our life. It becomes impossible to live without them. They influence our life one or other way. They are, especially in electronic media like TV, powerful tools to change consumers' behavior. The advertisers design and project materials in most attractive way to influence the viewers to feel good & instantly associate their feelings with the products. All promotional advertisements are meant for selling their products, though sometimes they are claimed to be educative. They do have hidden purpose, selling.

While the advertisement for common consumer items, if misleading, may cause loss of some money; the misleading and unethical advertisement on medicine can be dangerous. No modern medicine (in this respect medicine of any system) is absolutely safe. Every medicine is associated with some or other risk (side or unwanted effects of medicine). The common man does not have the full knowledge of the risk involved using the medicine. The advertisers always project the benefits and never the risk. The risk even if projected, they are written in such small letters that they are not readable.

Advertisements of medicines can be very misleading. Nothing works as good as consulting a doctor and getting a prescription.

The advertisement on medicines and diseases are controlled under Drugs and Magic Remedies (Objectionable Advertisement) Act. The Drugs and Cosmetics rules too specifies the diseases and ailments for which no claim to prevent or cure is available and hence advertisement for such diseases is prohibited. The disease oriented promotional campaign, often, present alarming figures on disease risk.

Direct to consumer advertisement on over the counter medicines may be educative and improve self-care practices. Such advertisements are permitted in many other countries also. Looking into our literacy and awareness level, the advertisement can be misleading to many as the advertisement too often does not give the details like: maximum dose, what precautions to be taken while taking the medicine, adverse reactions etc. Look into these few examples. An asthmatic or peptic ulcer patient may develop severe problems like precipitation of asthma or gastric bleeding if aspirin, a pain relief agent, is consumed. Alcoholics may further damage their livers if they continue taking Paracetamol, a pain and fever reducing medicine.

The advertisement on prescription drugs to the consumers is neither ethical nor legal. These medicines are permitted for sale only under the prescription of doctors. Even advertisements on such drugs are sometimes directly targeted to the consumers endangering their health to risk.

Medicines are aggressively advertised to induce consumption and self-medication. They are promoted as a way of obtaining happiness; with television ads making response to drugs appear instantaneous and magical. The consumers should be careful of such advertisements. What they need is better access to independent information in order to make informed choice. They need to know both benefits and risk involved in the use of drug treatment and non-drug treatment options, in additions to cost.

CHAPTER 33

Internet Medicines (e-Medicines)

In the IT era, everyone in the modern world has access to internet (in short net). It may be difficult to find people who have no knowledge of net. Net surfing becomes a routine as reading newspaper or listening television news every day. The internet is a global web connecting millions of computers in most countries throughout the world. Since the first launching of world wide web (www) in 1992, it has exploded into the mainstream culture. The web is a goldmine of information on just about any topic one can think of, and more are being added every day. As there is no regulation over the use of web, anyone can post information – accurate or inaccurate, helpful or misleading.

One can find a lot of information on health, diseases and medicines in the net. *No doubt that internet is a valuable source of information, but be sure to know and trust the source.*

One even finds offers of "medicine sale" in the net, sometimes claiming for curing ailments for which no cure is available. Buying medicines from other countries via internet is illegal. A line of caution - "Before using such medicine(s), consult your health care professionals". It may risk your health and cause waste of your money.

The medicines that are offered for sale may not be approved for use in our country. The country of origin may have poor regulations and the medicines get into market without rigorous trial to test safety and efficacy. The quality of such medicines cannot be assured. If a consumer experiences any hazard, it may not be possible to claim compensation, as the identity and source of location of such medicines cannot be established.

Look for authentic sites for medicine related information.
Do not buy medicines in internet.

The product of the same name (especially brand name) may contain different components in different countries. Lack of such awareness will lead to buying a wrong product.

The medicines that are offered for sale may be fraudulent. Treatment with such products may not only be just ineffective, but may be harmful to health. Sometimes it could be wasting your resources, valuable time and money.

Our country has clear regulations for importing medicines. The status of medicines whether medicine or OTC varies from country to country. If the particular medicine is not approved in our country, it may not be permitted to reach you by custom officials. Finally you get frustrated.

Appropriate medication or appropriate medical treatment for your disease is important for your health. Medicines cause harm if not properly used and some require to be used under direct supervision of doctors.

Reliable, truthful health or medical information is useful for the consumers to take informed decisions but are not the substitute to medical advice given by doctors.

The information that one gets in net is to be verified by finding out the source of information. The information site run by government organizations, institutions, voluntary associations etc., can be trusted while the web sites of individuals need to be scrutinized. Be careful sending money to buy medicine or even other products. Always counter check the information with another source to verify the authenticity.

CHAPTER 34

Medicine Information Sources (Where to Get Information)

One of the readers of my column from Bhubaneswar sent a post card seeking information on anti - epilepsy medicines. This further confirmed my belief that the consumers are in need of information on the medicines they are using. However, I am sure many of them may not know the source for seeking information or whom to ask for information they need, beside doctors and pharmacists. The present article is aimed at guiding the common public (including health professionals!) how should they obtain or seek information on medicines. The medicine information helps the consumers to understand the basic issues about medicines and help them learn how to use medicines safely and effectively.

The knowledge about medicines is constantly changing. More and more new medicines are made available for use in the market. More information on existing medicines too appears. It is essential that the doctors keep up to date knowledge on medicines they are prescribing. If a medicine induced illness occurs which the doctor could have known or prevented, courts in many countries would hold the doctor liable. Lack of knowledge is not an excuse. The other health care professionals and the consumers too need to know about the medicines they are handling or using for promoting appropriate use of the medicines.

Besides your doctor and pharmacist, the independent and institution based drug information centres are good sources of information.

There are many sources of medicine information ranging from standard books and journals to internet. Some are commercial and others are non-commercial. The drug companies too provide information as package inserts. The medicine information supplied by drug companies are reported to very often emphasize only on positive aspects of their product and overlook or give little coverage to the negative aspects. In simple sense, the drug companies' information may be biased. Non-commercial and independent source of medicine information is usually unbiased. The independent and unbiased medicine information to doctors, other health care professionals and the consumers is a prerequisite for improving the use of medicines.

Like many other countries, we too have independent medicine or drug information centres. The medicines information centre is a new concept for our country. The pharmacy institutions offering masters programme (M. Pharm.) in pharmacy practice (clinical pharmacy) have established drug information centers with both off line and on line references. These are usually hospital based. Other than these educational institutions, there are few independent, and not associated with the hospital, medicine information centres. These centres are exclusive for providing medicine and related information to everyone who approaches and are free too. The centres are well equipped with latest standard textbooks, journals, CD ROMs and on line facilities. They do provide service through e. mail and telephone. They do also publish Newsletters, which provide lots of information on medicines and their use in simple and user friendly way. There are around 20 drug information centers in the country inclusive of both hospitals based and independent. Here are the few independent and non-commercial drug information centers; list is not exhaustive:

Name of center and Location	Web site	e. mail address
Drug Information Centre of Karnataka State Pharmacy Council, Bangalore.	www.kspcdic.com	kspcdic@hotmail.com / kspcdic@blr.vsnl.net.in
Drug Information Centre of Maharastra State Pharmacy Council, Mumbai.	www.mspcindia.org/dic	dicmspc@yahoo.co.in / dicmspc@hathway.com
Indian Pharmaceutical Association, Bengal Branch	www.ipabengal.org	ipabengal.dic@gmail.com
Drug Information Centre of Tamil Nadu Pharmaceutical Welfare Trust, Chennai	www.pictrust.com	pictrust@hotmail.com

The National Human Rights Commission has already recommended to the government for establishment of computerized drug information center in all large hospitals. Once these recommendations are implemented the information would be available in your own locality. Till then, the interested person may directly contact the above listed independent centers, preferably through e. mails to get information on medicine and medicine use. This would not only help them how to use the medicines effectively and most appropriately but also protect them from ill effects of medicines to the extent possible.

CHAPTER 35

Patenting of Medicine

The government of India's patent ordinance is the New Year gift (2005) to the country's fellow men. With this country has temporarily complied with World Trade Organization's patent regulation. Under the new provision, the medicines/pharmaceuticals henceforth comes under product patent. India looses the advantage of process patent.

Patent provision in our country is regulated by Patent Act 1970 and Rules 1972. Patents are granted to the innovator/inventor to protect inventions from being copied and offer opportunity to recover the resources spent and make profit. Till now only process patents were allowed. The economists and industries that favour product patent urge that the provision would improve spending on R&D, encourage direct foreign investment leading to prosperity of the country. With the new provision, a patent holder will have exclusive manufacturing and marketing rights of invented new medicines for as long as 20 years.

Taking advantage of process patent provision, the pharmaceutical companies were at liberty to manufacture the medicine by other process or methods and market the same drug. This used to encourage market competition leading to reduce and stabilize price at an affordable level benefiting the Indian consumers. This is one of the reasons for having medicine prices in our country at one of the lowest in the world. The effort of CIPLA Company that made AIDS medicines available to the lesser-developed nations at an affordable rate is the classic example of importance of process patent in our national law. The multinationals were forced to bring down their AIDS drugs internationally.

As development of new drug is a time consuming and high resource spending events, it is doubtful that how many Indian Pharma companies can compete with multinationals.

Though patenting encourages innovation, patenting brings monopoly with increased prices of medicines.

Industry sources claim only about 3% of the existing drugs will continue to be in patent period. Many companies, who have been manufacturing these drugs taking advantage of process patent provision, will have to stop marketing such products. This is likely to cause scarcity of such drugs in the market and as innovator is the only marketer, the prices of such drugs would be higher.

The biggest fear is the price rise of medicines especially new ones. The prices of existing drugs still under patent would also go up. Even the price regulating mechanism (Drugs Price Control Order) of the government will fail to provide relief to the ailing citizens.

With unlimited resources at the disposal of multinationals and big Pharma companies, they would impress upon the doctors one or other way to prescribe their products available at higher price. Having prescribed the consumers will have no other options except to buy even at their inconvenience. The consumers need to be proactive and must ask the doctor whether cheaper alternatives available and go for it, if they wish to safe guard their pocket.

CHAPTER 36

Patent Medicine–Battle Finally Won!

The seven year long battle is finally won by India! The Supreme Court's ruling on 01st April against challenge of the Swiss multinational pharmaceutical company, Novartis, is a public victory. Novartis has been challenging the provision of Indian Patent Act arguing for patent of its anti-cancer drug, Glivec. The Supreme Court dismissing the petition of Novartis upheld the public health provision of Indian Patent Act benefiting millions of patients not only in India but around the globe.

While amending the Patent Act to comply with the obligations of World Trade Organization (WTO), the Indian Parliament kept a provision under section 3(d) of the Act as a public health measure to safeguard the interest of poor patients against the misuse of patents. The section 3(d) restricts patents for already known drugs unless the new claims are superior in efficacy. The pharma companies have been trying to extend the patent of their patented molecules by making slight and trivial changes to the existing original molecule. Glivec is chemically imatinib mesylate and is an excellent drug for leukemia, commonly called blood cancer. The imatinib mesylate is the salt form of the original molecule, imatinib. This is known as Gleevec in USA.

The Supreme Court observed that the original patent application filed in USA in 1994 had covered the imatinib mesylate as well as imatinib. In India, Novartis Pharma was trying to get patent for the beta crystalline variety of imatinib mesylate. Against the Novartis claim "Better physico-chemical qualities such as shape of the molecule, flowability, hygroscopicity and solubility satisfy the test for enhanced efficacy", the Supreme Court clarified "Physico-chemical properties of beta crystalline form of imatinib mesylate with improved flow properties, decreased hygroscopicity, and improved thermodynamic stability may be beneficial to the patients but they do not meet the standard of efficacy as required under section 3(d). This new form of Glivec has patent in many countries including USA, Russia and China.

Novartis first patented imatinib in 1994. Once India signed WTO's Trade Related Intellectual Property Rights (TRIPS) agreement, it had applied for patent for mesylate salt form of imatinib in 1998 at Chennai Patent Office. The patent office rejected the application based on section 3(d) of Patent (Amendment) Act 2005. Novartis then approached the Madras High Court challenging the decision of Chennai patent office and questioned the provision of the section. The Madras High Court rejected the Novartis challenge in 2007 but referred the case to the Intellectual Property Appellate Board (IPAB), which in turn rejected the application. The rejected Novartis finally approached Supreme Court of the country in 2009 and the Supreme Court finally dismissed Novartis's challenge. Dismissing the petition with cost the Supreme Court clarified that applicants of patent have to meet the standards of section 3(d) of Indian Patent Act before they can get the patent under Indian Law".

At the time when Novartis got the patent in 1994 in USA, there was no product patent in India and hence, no patent was made available in India. This led to generic version of the molecule in the market reducing the treatment cost substantially. The generic products were made available at less than one-tenth of Novartis's price. The beta crystalline salt of the molecule is claimed to have improved bioavailability and such changes in old molecule is patentable in USA and Europe, often called ever greening patenting. Had the new beta crystalline form got a patent in India, the company's monopoly for marketing would be another 20 years and a big market as there would be no generic supply from India. Currently the cost of treatment of blood cancer with this generic version is Rs. 8000 per month while the cost with Novartis product would be Rs. 1.2 Lakh per month.

In spite of international pressure, the Government has kept some provisions open in the best interest of countries ailing communities: not allowing ever greening of patent and compulsory licensing.

While the Supreme Court's judgment is welcomed worldwide, the critics have their own logic, but are unjustified. The critics say "India has killed medical innovation". Drug development is risky, requires enormous resources and progress comes step by step with one incremental innovation at a time. This incremental innovation too deserves patent. If no patent, no profit and no investment! No investment means no new drug. Without patent protection, an innovator company may not earn back the invested amount in Research and Development. It is also argued that this is not going to help the poor as more than 85% of Indian patients have been provided free Glivec.

While free Glivec is made available for only around 16,000 patients, there are more than 3 lakh patients who sustains due to generic cheaper versions. There are around reported to be 28 lakh cancer patients in the country. The investment of Novartis on Glivec is claimed to be not substantial as the company received orphan drug tax credit, small size of the clinical trial and its short development time. Its first clinical trial took place in June 1998 and obtained marketing approval in 10th May 2001.

But this was not just the case of Glivec alone and the judgment will have affect on many more drugs. This would facilitate early entry of generic medicines into the market for many other medicines. Earlier India rejected the patents of ant-HIV drugs on the grounds of mere modifications. The whole world has been closely watching this case as the judgment has remarkable impact on the access to medicines to millions and millions of patients living in India and similar developing countries. Had Novartis won, it would have made provision for ever greening patents in India like USA and that would have provided patent for the new form with 20 years monopoly to market the medicine at a price of its choice. Now the judgment would prevent other companies approaching India for similar patents and India would continue to manufacture and supply low cost generic versions benefiting people worldwide.

This is a victory on rights of the patients on access to affordable quality medicines over the patent monopoly of pharma companies. Though Novartis has option to file review petition against the judgment within 90 days, let's hope the good sense would prevail and Novartis would respect the judgment and sentiments of the people.

CHAPTER 37

Use, Misuse and Abuse of Medicines

While evaluating a paper of a student appeared in practical examination, I noticed that he has completed all the pages writing the questions repeatedly. On enquiry he revealed that he did not sleep in the previous night preparing for examination. He had taken some medicines to keep himself awake throughout night. He was fully satisfied with his answers, but in reality it was otherwise. This is a classical case of medicine misuse. He used medicine for mental stimulation and to improve confidence, but his performance was nil.

Though it is difficult to distinguish the use, misuse and abuse terminology, they may be simplified as follows: The use of medicines for appropriate medical purpose is termed as use. The medicines are useful alleviating sufferings. Some medicines, while very useful often used for non-medical purpose. The misuse refers to inappropriate use of legal medicines intended to be medications. Abuse is referred to any use of legal or illegal medicines (or, drugs) when it is detrimental for health and well-being. The use of medicines or similar substances for non-medical purpose is abuse.

Drug misuse is also alarming and life threatening. Misuse may occur when a patient misunderstands the direction for use of a prescription or non-prescription medicine or when a patient shares his or her medicines with friend or family members for whom the medicine was not prescribed or intended. The use of medicine for a purpose or condition other than that for which it is intended or at a dosage other than that recommended is also misuse. Sometimes the mis-user is lucky and no adverse reactions occur. On occasion misuse practice can have tragic consequences.

The medicines that are abused are usually called drugs (illegal substances) and while terminology medicines (legally approved for use) are reserved when they are for medical use, though there is no clear-cut distinction. Drug abuse is a clear danger to the society. The cost of drug abuse to the individual are extensive and include absenteeism, underachievement, loss of job, marital instability, loss of self esteem, serious illness and even death. Drug abuse not only causes dependence, they too cause increase of risk of HIV and Hepatitis C infection if many share syringe. There is a serious withdrawal problem. The drugs most often associated with abuse are psychoactive or mind altering drugs.

Medicines are meant for useful purpose. Their misuse and abuse must be avoided in the best interest of individual's health and society as a whole.

The problem associated with drug misuse or abuse in our society extends beyond the illegal drugs. Though there is misuse or abuse of social drugs like alcohol, nicotine and caffeine, the present article intends to educate the public on danger of prescription and OTC medicines being misused and abused.

The misuse and abuse of medicines are dangerous. Misuse of medicines like taking too much, not finishing a course, etc., may cause toxic effects or resistance. The most frequently abused categories of medicines include: Opioids, stimulants and sedatives. Opiods are narcotics typically used for relieving pain included morphine, codeine and derivatives. The stimulants affect central nervous system and increase mental alertness, decrease fatigue and produce a sense of well-being. Amphetamine comes under this category. Sedatives depress the central nervous system and are frequently used to treat anxiety, panic disorder, and sleeplessness. Barbiturates and diazepam type of medicines fall in this type. Initially these medicines are used for medical purpose and latter become the substance of abuse. Even cough syrups can cause addiction like above medicines. Use leads to abuse.

The use and abuse of medicines occur in all income and education levels, among all ethnic groups and at all ages. But the young and teenagers are most vulnerable. Initially they start using drugs for fun and enjoyment. But quickly do they realize that they are duped and life has become unmanageable without drugs.

The medicines are for medical purpose and they should be used appropriately for best results. The abuse of medicines can be a threat to society. Abuse leads to addiction and dependence. Life becomes miserable without drugs. The treatment of addiction is available and there are several de-addicting centers supported by governments. Prevention of abuse is the responsibility of many including doctors and the patients as well. But it is the patients or public who are affected and they must take firm decision about their life, even in the face of peer pressure. Simply all you need to say is "No for such Drugs for pleasure" and protect your life from the adverse affects of drug abuse.

CHAPTER 38

Use and Abuse of Medicines in Sports

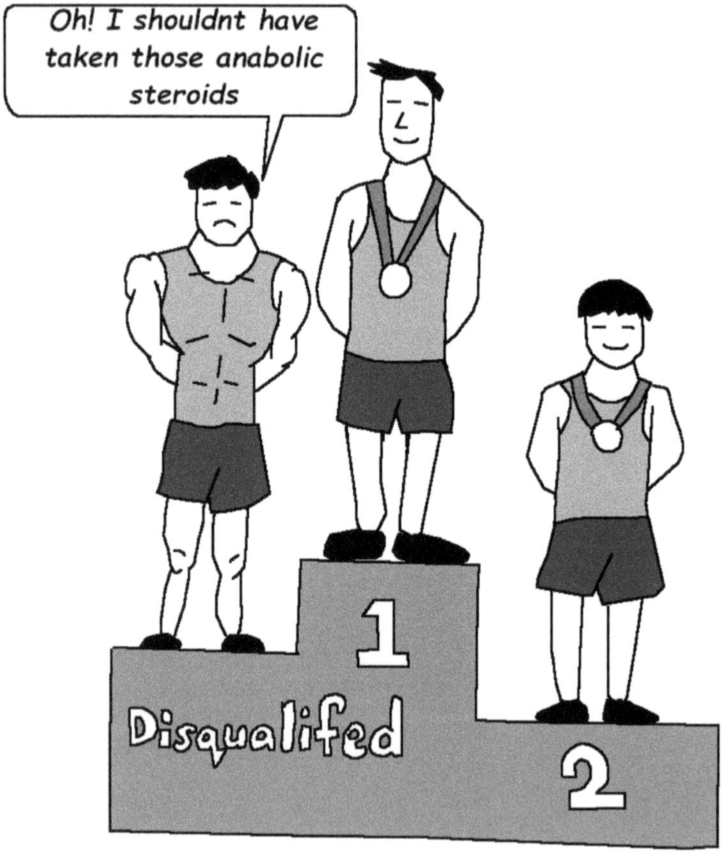

India was fourth in medal tally in the recently held 18th Commonwealth games in Melbourne, Australia. But the occasion of celebration was marked with both glory and shame. The two weight lifters were tested positive for anabolic steroids. In a competitive world of sports, the athletes are continually on the lookout for a winning edge; often they look for medicines for improving performance.

As early as in 300 BC, Greek athletes were reported to have taken hallucinogenic mushrooms to improve performance in competition. In modern era, the drugs have continued to be a factor in athletic competition. In post world war II, many new body building drugs (anabolic steroids) based on male sex hormone, testosterone, were introduced and naturally the athletes, coaches and trainers were all interested. The anabolic steroids promote masculine changes in the body and increased muscular development. The events requiring strength and size, anabolic steroids were seen to be perfectly suited for gaining competitive advantage. For the first time in the history of sports, in September 1988 in Seol Olympic games, Canadian sprinter Ben Johnson was denied the gold medal despite of achieving the 100 meter dash in world record breaking time of 9.79 seconds because he was tested positive for anabolic steroids. The world started realizing the pervasiveness of this practice of using drugs and cheating in sports.

The most common symptom of use of anabolic steroid is a dramatic increase in body bulk. The users feel more energetic and often have an increased sexual desire. The side effects are dose dependent. Erratic mood swings, irrational behaviors, increased aggressiveness are common problems at high doses. Acne gets worse. Jaundice may occur if user has liver damage.

In a competitive world of sports, the athletes are in continuing look out for winning edge, often they look for medicines for improving performance. The use of medicines for improving performance in sports is illegal.

Though there have been efforts to develop screening procedure to prevent the use of drugs from resulting in one competitor having an unfair advantage over another. The drug testing procedure usually involves collection of urine from the individual and analyzed using sophisticated analytical techniques for presence of drugs or their metabolites. The commercial testing kit is available for screening major controlled substances (opiates, amphetamine, cocaine, benzodiazepines, marijuana). The blood sample is also analyzed for screening. This drug testing is called doping. The word dope originates from the practice of Kaffir tribesmen in South Africa who drank a mixture of alcohol and cola called dop, to gain increased energy and stamina. Later the 'e' is added to make it dope.

The World Anti Doping Agency (WADA) usually monitors the use and abuse of medicines in sports. It publishes an international standard list each year of prohibited substances and methods. The current world anti doping code can be obtained from its website: www.wada-ama.org.

Finasteride (androgen synthesis inhibitor used prostate cancer, male pattern baldness) is prohibited during and out of competition because the alpha – reductase inhibitors are considered potential masking agents for drug testing. Use of beta – 2 agonists such as salbutamol inhaler is also in the prohibited list. Certain herbal and nutritional products may contain banned substance such as ephedrine in Chinese ephedra.

Prohibited substances (in and out of competition)

1. Anabolic steroids like nandrolone and stanozolol.
2. Hormones and related substances such as erythropoietin.
3. Beta-2 agonists such as salbutamol, terbutaline etc.
4. Agents with anti-estrogenic activity such as tamoxifen and clomiphene.
5. Diuretics and other masking agents like acetazolamide, spironolactone etc.

Prohibited substances (in competition only)

1. Stimulants like amphetamine, cocaine etc.
2. Narcotics like pethidine, pentazocine etc.
3. Cannabinoids such as hashish and marijuana.
4. Glucocorticoids.

(Please note that the list is not exhaustive)

While it is essential that efforts need to be made to enhance performance, but should be done under the legal guidelines of WADA. Sports persons and athletes should be aware of banned medicines during competitions and discuss with their doctors or coaches before taking even simple cough and cold remedies.

CHAPTER 39

Splitting of Tablets

Tablets are the most convenient, popular and cheapest medicinal products. Often it is recommended or prescribed to take half of a tablet as dose. The patient needs to split (or break) the tablets into two equal halves and take half tablet as one dose.

The prime reason for tablet splitting is to obtain the required strength (dose) for the individual. Sometimes the required strength of tablet may not be available commercially. The commercially available strength product may not be suitable. The usual dose as mentioned on label or as recommended by product manufacturer may not be suitable for every one. Exact dose is necessary to avoid unnecessary adverse effects of medicines. Patient's exact requirement may be more than one tablet or fraction of a tablet. The liquid preparations may not be available for stability or other reasons or may be costly. Usually elderly patients or children require reduced dose. In such situations, it is necessary to buy or get a higher strength tablet(s) and break to take ½ (or even ¼ tablet) per dose.

Patients face several problems in splitting tablets. The patients suffering from arthritis, parkinsonism and elderly may not have the visual acuity or manual strength to break the tablets evenly. Split tablets often crumble easily and thus difficult to handle. Patients often get confused and split wrong medicines or even get tired of splitting and ultimately stop taking medicines.

The splitting of tablets leads to inaccuracy in dosing. Correct dosing is necessary for therapeutic effect and to avoid unnecessary adverse effects. The splitting is discouraged.

Uneven breaking of tablets may result in significant fluctuations in the dose. This is particularly true with high potency medicines (low dose medicines). There is even possibility of unequal distribution of active drug within the tablet as large proportions of inert materials are included to make tablets. The split tablets get degraded prematurely as they are out of package (blister or strip). They often differ in their performance too compared to intact tablets.

Small size, unusually thick, irregularly shaped, un-scored or scored in one side only tablets, if split, unlikely to have accurate breaking into two halves. The tablets scored on both sides are usually considered suitable for division, but some even may not break easily.

Tablets can be split into two portions by either breaking with fingers along a scored line or cutting with a knife. Uneven breaking not only causes inaccurate dose but may increase wastage too. The tablets may crumble or break into more than two parts. Patients often split number of tablets in advance for convenience. The environmental exposure of broken tablets to air and light may affect the stability of the medicinal ingredient. A classic example is Aspirin tablets. The broken tablets become unsuitable for use later as aspirin hydrolyses on exposure to environmental moisture. If only half of the tablet is to be taken as dose, the unused fraction of the tablet needs to be thrown out immediately.

Certain categories of tablets: coated tablets, sustained release tablets are not suitable for splitting. The tablets are coated for several reasons: to mask the taste (sugar coating), to protect against environmental hazards and /or to by-pass stomach (enteric coating). On breaking the coating gets damaged and the purpose or benefit of coating is lost. Similarly the sustained release tablets are designed for a purpose to achieve long duration of action from single dose. The design would be damaged on breaking. These categories of tablets are not meant for splitting and using the fraction of tablet as dose.

The patients need to remember the following tips if advised for splitting of tablets:

- Insist on appropriate strength of tablets if commercially available. Use liquid products for easy dose adjustment. Splitting of tablets is not the safest option available for dose adjustment, if specific dose is available commercially.
- Check the product type: Enteric coated/sugar coated or sustained release tablets are not suitable for splitting. Pre-packed oral contraceptives are not intended for splitting.

- Scored tablets are only recommended for splitting.
- Learn the appropriate storage of split tablets. They may get decomposed on exposure to moisture and light on environment.
- Wash and wipe your hand (to make dry) before splitting tablets.
- If you have difficulty in splitting, never hesitate to take someone's help in the family.

CHAPTER 40

Use of Injections

I remember reading a newspaper report that the child was amputed of her hand because of wrong administration of injection. The intravenous injection was wrongfully given through an artery leading ultimately loosing hand. This is just one type of complication or problem associated with injection practice or use. There are many. It is essential that the people should be aware of when to use injection and when to avoid.

Injections are just another method or route of medicines' administration similar to tablets and capsules. The effects of medicines are similar whether they are given by oral or injection route except few exceptions. Though injections provide quick relief (not always), it is not desirable to have injection for each and every health problem. There are several types of injections: intravenous, subcutaneous, intra dermal, intra muscular, intra arterial etc. The types of medicine and the medical need decide the route of injection.

The injections are normally advised or indicated in the following conditions: the medicine is available only in this form (as it may not be practicable or feasible to administer by other route, like insulin), patient is unable to use other form like tablets, capsules or liquids (in unconscious, vomiting and in emergency), when immediate effect is desired (like severe asthma, severe dehydration etc.). The injections too offer unique opportunity for dose adjustment and sometimes administration of several medicines simultaneously, useful in critically ill patients.

There are several drawbacks associated with injection use. Skilled and knowledgeable person is necessary for giving injection. Self-administration is not possible except for injection of insulin where patients are trained for it. Almost every one of us has fear of needle prick and the children sometimes develop phobia for going to hospital out of fear. Too rapid of injection could be hazardous in some cases. If person administering is unaware of this fact, could lead to severe complications.

Injection of aminophylline (in asthma), adrenaline and iron come under this category. Accidental over dosing cannot be easily treated. Thrombosis or tissue irritation is common at injection site.

Use injection when other methods of use are not feasible or in emergency. Destroy the disposable syringe and needle to prevent getting recycled.

As all injections use needle to pierce the skin, there is always a risk of viral or bacterial infection, if injection is not sterile or appropriate sterilization practice is not followed. Drug abusers too use injections as they get rapid and intense effect. They very often share the same needle and syringe causing further risk of transferring infections from one to the other. There are reports of polio caused by injections. However, at present the biggest threat is risk of getting infected with hepatitis and HIV (AIDS) from sharing or using the contaminated needle. The recycled disposable syringe or needle is common. Even, sometimes, in clinic or hospital same needle is used for several patients. This practice is dangerous. The proper disposal of used needle and syringe is essential, failing which the rag pickers collect them and these get re-circulated with a fresh pack even without sterilization.

Many injections advised by health professionals are not only unnecessarily dangerous, but are inconvenient too to the patients. The injection forms of medicines are costlier and the total treatment cost is much higher compared to using medicines in oral form. Just with profit motive or for generating more revenue, they are prescribed. One needs to be vigilant and make sure that the injection is essential for treatment. Here are few simple guidelines for safe injection practice:

- Do ask your doctor or health professional who advises injection, whether alternate to it is available or feasible. It is your right. You are more concerned to your well being than any body's else.
- You must tell your doctor that you do not have facility or person who can administer the injection. He would appropriately advise.
- Tell your doctor or nurse who administers injection, if you are allergic to it. If you are not sure, insist on sensitivity testing before full injection. Some injections like penicillin, anti-snake venom etc., can cause serious life threatening reaction like anaphylactic shock on injection.

- Be sure that sterilized injection set is used at each injection. The needle and syringe can be sterilized at home by boiling for at least 30 minutes or by steaming in domestic pressure cooker (15 minutes after first whistle). Do not touch the tip of the needle it may get contaminated again.
- Insist on sterilizing the skin surface before injection either by use of spirit or any other disinfectant.
- Destroy the disposable injection sets so that they would no longer be possible for re-circulation. Bury or break them.
- Remember, the injections are more troublesome and dangerous too than oral medicines.

CHAPTER 41

Jan Aushadhi for Affordable Quality Medicines

Undoubtedly the medicines are one of the most important components of the healthcare delivery system perhaps next to the health professionals. But unfortunately the statistics shows that two third of India's population lack access to essential medicines against the world average one third population without access to essential medicines (World Medicine Situation 2004). The National Sample Survey (Morbidity Survey) of 2004 showed that the medicines account for 81% of household health care expenditure in rural areas and 75% in urban areas with an average figure of 79%. As the share of expenditure on medicine in total expenditure on health care is higher among the poor, undoubtedly one of the main reasons for lack of access is price of medicines.

Realizing the price of the medicines (affordability) as one of the important determining factor for improving access to medicines, the Department of Pharmaceuticals, Government of India, initiated the operation of Peoples' medicines shop, called Jan Aushadhi, all over the country. These shops are aimed to sell generic medicines only at much cheaper rate than the price of corresponding branded medicines. The first such store has been opened at Amritsar with cooperation of Punjab government. Besides Punjab the other states like Rajasthan and Orissa have already started these stores for the benefit of the public. To cite an example of the price of the medicines sold in the Jan Aushadhi, the price of 10 tablets of Ciprofloxacin costs Rs. 20.10 in January 2009 against the price of the branded product of same10 tablets was Rs. 97.00. This shows that the medicines would be made available at a much discounted price in these stores.

It has been reported that there are apprehensions on establishment of Jan Aushadhi in Government Hospitals in Tamil Nadu as it might affect poor patients' right to get quality medicines free of cost. One needs to look into the whole scheme which is basically meant to offer quality medicines at affordable prices. The medicines available at these stores are not cheap alternatives to branded products. They are just affordable quality medicines.

Coming to the quality of medicines, there is no second quality. All medicines available in the market are expected to comply with the quality parameters specified in the pharmacopoeias. The pharmacopoeias are book of standards for medicines. There are regulations to control. All manufacturers are required to have Good Manufacturing Practice Standards for making medicines. Even it is not possible to distinguish between a product that comply with standard (quality product) and a product that does not comply with the standard (not a quality product) unless laboratory investigation is done. There are reports too on many branded products not complying with quality parameters specified in pharmacopoeias.

Jan Aushadhi or similar generic medicine stores established by various agencies provide good opportunity to buy quality medicines at affordable prices.

While brand and generics often have different meaning in different countries, in India when medicines are sold by common name (International Non-Proprietary Name (INN)), then they are called generics. There are lots of myths about generic medicines.

Sl. No.	Myth	Fact
1	Generic medicines cost less because they are inferior.	Generic manufacturers are able to sell their products at lower prices, not because the products are of lower quality, but because they do not engage in costly advertising, marketing or promotion or research and development.
2	People who are switched to a generic drug are risking treatment failure.	Treatment failure can and do occur with both generic or brand name drugs.
3	Generics take longer to act in the body.	The firm seeking to sell a generic drug must show that its drug delivers the same amount of active ingredient in the same time frame as the original product.
4	Generics are not as potent as brand-name drugs.	Drugs Control Authority ensures that all products available in the market met the specified criteria in terms of quality, strength, purity and stability. No separate rule exists either for branded or generics.

Table *Contd...*

Sl. No.	Myth	Fact
5	Brand names drugs are safer than generic drugs.	Adverse drug reactions are basically dependent on active drug component. Hence ADR can occur in both cases.
6	Drugs Control Authorities do not care about concerns over generic drugs.	There is same protocol for approval of products whether in brand or generic name.
7	As the Doctors prescribe brand names they must be superior.	Just by name or packaging of product, it is not possible to distinguish between good product and substandard product. Neither the doctor nor the chemist can differentiate without laboratory checking. The doctors prescribe in brands because of aggressive marketing or promotion of brands by the respective companies.
8	Branded products have no counterfeiting. Generics do have. Hence opting for generics may lead to buying counterfeit medicines.	Counterfeits are found for both brands and generics. It is difficult to check.

The use of generics is not just promoted in poor or developing countries. The use of generics is encouraged throughout the world including UK, USA, The Netherlands, Sweden, Denmark etc. In fact, the World Health Organization advocates the use of generic medicines for reducing the healthcare costs. The study showed that in USA 68% of the prescriptions are filled with generic products in 2008 against 50% of the prescriptions filled with generics in 2003. This clearly shows the world trend towards generics.

The Jan Aushadhi Stores are not meant for poor alone. Others too can buy medicines from these stores which would help them not only saving their hard earned money but would also ensure quality. As these stores are managed by Self Help Group or Non-Government Organizations (NGOs), chances of dealing with spurious drugs are too remote. They are not meant to be an alternative to free supply of medicines at government health facilities. Jan Aushadhi is for everyone. They even need to be established in busy town area to serve more number of people.

CHAPTER 42

Off Label Use of Medicines (Pill Poppers, Wake Up!)

The Food and Drug Administration (FDA) of USA, one of the most respected drug regulatory bodies in the world, recently warned against the use of quinine to treat leg cramps. The quinine is an approved anti-malarial medicine with a narrow margin between an effective dose and toxic dose. As malaria is life threatening, the use of quinine is justified despite the risk involved. On the other hand because of its serious side effects including death, it should not be used to prevent or treat leg cramps. The use of quinine in treating leg cramps is called 'off label use'. The use of an approved medicine for other than the intended indication (approved use) is known as 'off label use'.

The off label use of medicines is not new. It is common throughout the world. The study showed that the doctors are often ignorant of meaning of off label use. The pharmaceutical companies market their products sometimes for the unapproved indications. Though legally no unapproved drug is permissible to be marketed in the country, there is little legislative control for preventing off label use. An approved drug for certain claims (indications/use), if proposed to be marketed with modified or new claim (use) is treated as new drug in our legislation.

In couple of year back it was alleged that the pharmaceutical companies illegally promoted an anticancer medicine, letrozole, for improving fertility in females in India. The central government had warned the concerned pharmaceutical companies of such illegal and unethical practice of drug promotion. Letrozole is expensive anti-cancer medicine and known for its toxicity. It is also teratogenic and can cause malformation of babies.

The marketing approval of new drug is based on evidence collected during pre-clinical (animal study) and clinical study (clinical trial). Based on these studies, the dose, frequency, duration of treatment are determined for a particular use. The likely side effects during use for these conditions are also documented. When the same drug is tried for other indication or use, the above particulars too get changed. The dose, frequency, duration and possible side effects may differ. Hence full testing of the medicine for new indication is essential like as done at least in clinical trial.

Off Label use is unethical and illegal.

The safety and efficacy are the two important hallmarks of medicines. The physicians are expected to weigh the benefits of the medicines in treating disease (or the patient) against likely suffering by the patient (risks). The benefit /risk ratio is the determining factor for medication use. Off label use is often based on anecdotal data, but not on sound clinical evidence. Such off label prescribing practice is viewed as human experimentation. Here are few examples of medicines that have been reported to have been used in off label prescribing practice (at different times):

Medicine	Approved indication (or use)	Off label use
Terbutaline sulphate	To prevent and relief of bronchospasm	Delay or inhibition of labour during birth process (tocolysis)
Injection of corticosteroid	Various purposes	Periocular injection (injection to eyes)
Nesiritde	Congestive heart failure in inpatients	Used in outpatient clinics
Quinine	Anti-malaria	In leg cramps
Letrozole	Anti-cancer	For fertility in female
Thalidomide	Anti-leprosy	Multiple myeloma (cancer)
Cyproheptadine	Antihistamine	Appetite stimulant
Sildenafil	Erectile dysfunction	Paediatric cardiac problem

Off label use promotion makes more information available to physicians enabling them to make better treatment recommendations for the patients. It allows the pharma companies to avoid seeking approval from drug regulatory bodies and making the products available quickly. The off label prescribing practice is especially useful for treating orphan diseases for which limited number of medicines commercially available. On the other hand the off label use practice under cuts the drug regulatory bodies ability to ensure safety and efficacy. The patients are at receiving end.

Promoting the use of medicines for unapproved use is unlawful activity in our country. Under the Drugs and Cosmetics Act, if the label of the product or anything accompanying the product (medical literature/package inserts) makes a false or misleading claim, then such products are termed as misbranded. The prescribers are ethically responsible for informing the patients whenever they are prescribed medicines under off label use. The prescribers and the manufacturers can be held responsible under various provisions of laws including Consumers' Protection Acts for such illegal and unethical practices.

CHAPTER 43

Herbal Medicines

"Traditional Indian (Ayurvedic) and Chinese Medicines associated with heavy metal poisoning" is the head line of the current issue of Australian Adverse drug Reaction Bulletin (February 2007). Its report continues "A married couple who both showed elevated blood lead levels after taking Ayurvedic herbal medicines, dispensed from Indian hospital. The man was admitted to hospital in Australia with abdominal pain, nausea and vomiting secondary to lead poisoning. He had a lead level of 120 microgram per decilitre (120 mcg %) and also high levels arsenic and mercury. However, wife was asymptomatic but had high level of lead". This is not the first time the people or regulatory bodies of other countries suspect the quality of Indian system of medicines. The Indian herbal medicines are reported to even contain synthetic steroids. Another report from Madras Diabetes Research Foundation claimed to have experienced at least three deaths due to patients resorting herbal cures for diabetes.

In spite of spectacular advances in modern medicine including genetic engineering, biotechnology, organ transplant, designer drugs etc., a large number of population in many countries including India rely on herbal and other complimentary medicines for primary health care. Herbal medicines are common to all races and cultures. Dating from time immemorial, it has been in practice throughout the world. Indian Ayurvedic system of medicine is predominately based on herbs. No one has doubt regarding the usefulness of herbal medicines. The World Health Organization (WHO) defines herbal medicines as plant derived materials or preparations with therapeutic or health benefits. They may contain either raw or processed ingredients from one or other plants. They are now available in a dosage forms similar to modern system of medicines.

While the medicines of modern systems have undergone strict procedures of screening or testing before getting approval as medicines, the herbal systems do not have such regulation requirements. Though allopathic (modern) medicines are brought under regulation of the government in 1940, the Ayurvedic, Sidha and Unani system of medicines were kept out of control. They have been included for regulation only in 1964 under Drugs and Cosmetics Act. At present the Indian legislation controls the import, export, manufacture and sale of these medicines. However no sale licence is necessary, provided the medicines are manufactured under a valid licence. In order to improve the quality of herbal medicines (including medicines of Ayurvedic medicines), the government of India has introduced the concept of Good Manufacturing Practice (GMP). Many companies have accepted this standard and many more are yet to comply. The GMP adoption though improve the quality of medicines, still it does not assure unless full quality assurance programme is implemented. Quality assurance programme is a part of medicines' manufacturing system of modern medicines. It is necessary to have similar programmes for herbal medicines too. The small manufacturing units and individuals often have difficulties in implementing GMP and other quality requirements because of several constraints. There are practical difficulties too. The herbal medicines often contain several herbs together and each with several chemical components.

Chinese herbal medicines are more popular than the similar medicines of India. This is because we still rely on traditional values not on science. Like modern medicines, the world needs to have evidence of safety and efficacy of herbal medicines. The efficacy is time tested but no evidence of record of its safety (means no toxicity). Many randomised controlled trials (RCT) have shown the evidence of herbal medicines' efficacy. RCTs are the foundation of evidence based medicine.

Herbal medicines often interact with modern medicines. You must tell your doctor what medicines you are taking. They too are very toxic especially those containing heavy metals.

When the heavy metal contents of Indian medicines are raised internationally, the government of India made the testing of medicines for heavy metal content is mandatory for medicines required for export. But for domestic consumption the manufacturer need not test them. Indians are different from people of other countries? Heavy metals are known to be toxic to all races.

People face some potential problems with use of herbal medicines: like unknowingly using suspect or counterfeit products; choosing inappropriate therapies in self care and unintentional over dosing. The unqualified practitioners or quacks further aggravate the situation. Indian rule does not allow an allopathic doctor to prescribe medicines of other system or vice versa. Another potential risk is that the patients do not inform their doctors about the use of similar medicines. The studies have shown that the mixing of herbal medicines and allopathic medicines can cause more harm than any one has realized. In one study it is reported that intake of St. John's wort, a top selling herb used to treat depression seemed to interfere with the action of cyclosporine, anti-rejection medicine to transplant patients. The interference in metabolism of the cyclosporine reduces its concentration resulting in reduced effect.

The medicines are meant for treating our illness, maintaining our health or preventing illness. They should be used with care and caution as they too can cause toxic effects or problems. Here are few rational guidelines for using herbal medicines:

- Do not believe blindly that the herbal medicines are from nature and they are safe and free of side effects.
- Is or are the products are from reputed licensed manufacturers. They are likely to have good quality assurance programmes.
- Check whether the medicines are suitable for your disease or condition.
- Use herbal medicines if they are prescribed by qualified practitioners only.
- Tell your allopathic doctor that you have been using herbal medicine (if any).
- Inform your doctor, if you experience any side effects or unusual effects after using the medicine.

PART B
Medicine Administration

CHAPTER 44

Orally Taking Medicines

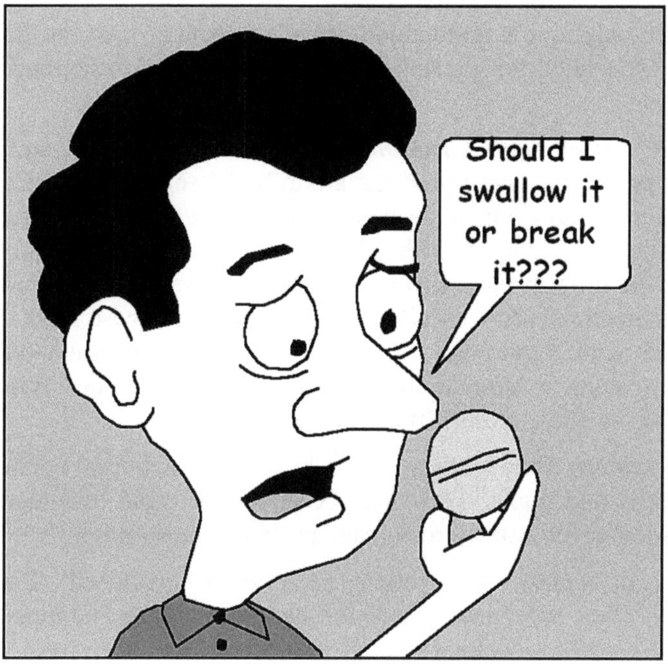

The appropriate use of the medicine is the key element in successful drug therapy. Understanding the use of medicines help the patients to use them safe and effectively.

Oral dosage forms are the safest, cheapest and commonest form of drug delivery. They are the first choice in medications. They are available in a variety of forms ranging from solids to liquids.

Tables and Capsules

***Swallowable tablets/capsules*:** They are to be swallowed with a tumbler of water. The water helps in dissolution, a primary requirement for drug absorption. Usually such products are to be swallowed as they are. "Swallow with sufficient water" is the instruction.

Water would also ensure passage of tablets/capsules into the stomach. The tablets/capsules, sometimes, get lodged within the esophagus, if not swallowed with sufficient water. Esophagus ulceration was reported due to lodging of drugs.

During night, it is preferable to swallow them at least one hour before retiring specially for patients suffering from gastro-esophageal reflux diseases.

***Enteric coated and sustained release/controlled release/extended release products*:** These products are to be taken/swallowed intact. They are never to be divided or broken before swallowing. Enteric-coated preparations are coated with materials that will by-pass stomach and release the drug through disintegration and dissolution in intestine only. The sustained release/controlled release/extended release products too are designed with a purpose to release drug at predetermined/controlled manner to achieve long duration effect. Patient need to be advised as "Do not break, swallow with sufficient water".

***Buccal tablets*:** They are intended to be kept in the buccal pouch between the cheeks and gums. They may be either for rapid disintegration and dissolution or for a slow erosion and prolonged absorption.

***Sublingual tablets*:** The patient need to be instructed "Place under tongue". There are many reasons for making sublingual administration: to improve/promote/accelerate drug absorption or to bypass first pass elimination.

***Dispersible/Effervescent tablets*:** The dispersible tablets are normally made for children. "Keep the tablet with little water in a spoon, allow it to mix and then give to child to swallow" is the instruction. Effervescent tablets are to be placed in water and to be taken while effervescing. The dispersible tablets are the alternative to liquid preparations and effervescent preparations offer a pleasant drink.

***Chewable tablets*:** They are designed to be chewed and then swallowed, but not to be swallowed intact. Chewing causes rapid disintegration for faster action. The patient is required to be instructed "Chew the tablet before swallowing".

Lozenges: They are designed to dissolve slowly to provide local effects in the oral cavity or pharynx (throat). They stimulate the production of oral secretions and provide a comforting and demulcent effect in minor throat or oral cavity irritations.

Oral Liquids

Suspension/emulsion: The patient should be advised on the need of shaking the bottle every time taking medicine. Instruction should be "Shake the bottle before measuring each dose". Shaking makes the preparation uniform. It would be inaccurate dosing if dose is measured without proper shaking.

Dose measurement: The dose measurement must be done with a measuring spoon. The domestic spoons vary widely in their capacity. Teaspoonful, tablespoonful terminology should be avoided. The liquid medicines must always be supplied with a measuring dose device. The calibrated droppers are to be supplied along with paediatric drops.

Mouthwashes and gargles: Both are concentrated solutions, usually, diluted with drinking water prior to use. Mouthwashes are used for oral hygiene and to treat infection of the mouth. They are also used as deodorant. They are not to be swallowed in large amounts.

Gargles are used to relieve soreness in mild throat infections. The gargling is done by holding the liquid in the throat and keeping in motion by a stream of air from the lungs. Like mouthwashes they too are not to be swallowed in large quantity. However, little accidental swallowing is harmless.

You may find the instruction as "Dilute one teaspoonful with half a tumbler of drinking water". "Do not swallow in large quantity" is another important instruction.

Linctuses: They are usually formulated with syrup as base to sooth sore mucous membranes in the treatment of cough. They have demulcent effect on the throat. They need to be swallowed slowly and undiluted to improve and prolong contact. "Swallow slowly without aid of water" should be the advice to patients.

Oral powders for reconstitution: These products are available as powders but to make into liquid forms (either solution or suspensions) before use. As some drugs exhibit limited chemical stability in liquid form, they are made available as powders for reconstitution. In general, they are needed to be stored in refrigerator and should be discarded after one/two weeks following reconstitutions as per manufacturer's instruction.

"Add boiled and cooled drinking water up to the mark on the bottle and shake to make uniform mixture" and "Shake every time before measuring dose" for suspensions are two important instructions.

CHAPTER 45

Ophthalmic Medicines

(a) Ophthalmic Medicines

Eyes are the most sensitive organs of the human body. A variety of drugs are applied to the eye for the localized effect of the medications on the surface of the eye or on its interior. The commonly used eye reparations include eye drops, eye ointments and eye lotions. However, recently ophthalmic inserts have also been introduced to provide for continuous release of medications. In this article, how these products are to be used is discussed briefly for the benefit of community pharmacists, which would help them counseling their patients on the use of eye preparations.

These preparations are sterile and the sterility is required to be maintained throughout the period of use.

Eye Drops: They are sterile solutions or suspensions intended to be instilled into the lower conjunctivital sac. They contain multiple dosages. Like oral suspensions, the suspension eye drops need to be shaken prior to use. They are supplied with drop administering device and usually packed in glass or plastic container. Some plastic packages contain a fixed, built in dropper that releases the medication when held in inverted position.

The patient must exercise care in protecting eye drops from contaminations. Drops packed with fixed dropper are less likely to acquire air borne contamination than the usual eye drops. However, each type is subject to contamination during use, brought about by touching of the tip of dropper to tissue or air borne contaminants.

Use one drop at a time. If second drop is necessary wait for few minutes before putting another drop.

The patient should be advised about the correct number of drops to instil. The capacity of the eye to retain the instilled fluid is limited. Most of the commercial eye drops deliver drop volume more than the retention capacity and thus much is lost through drainage. As the instilled volume increases, the rate of drainage increases, i.e., larger drops drain more rapidly. Smaller drops are more effective. If multiple drop therapy is desired, 5-minute interval between drops is recommended.

To allow the drop to remain in the eye and enhance efficiency, the patient should press his/her finger against the inner corner of the eye for 1 minute. This prevents the medication from entering tear duct. After instillation the patient should close his eye as long as possible, preferably 1-2 minutes and wipe any excess liquid off with a tissue.

If drops are applied or placed directly to the eye ball (cornea), they may cause a stinging sensation. They are instilled into the pocket formed by gentle pulling the eyelid. Once the drops have been instilled, the dropper should be returned to the original container and capped tightly. The dropper should not be rinsed or wiped off.

The instruction to patients follows:

1. Wash your hands.
2. Do not touch the dropper opening.
3. Look upward.
4. Pull the lower eyelid down to make a gutter.
5. Bring the dropper as close to the gutter as possible without touching it or the eye.
6. Apply the prescribed amount of drops.
7. Close the eye for about 10 minutes. Do not shut the eyes too tight.
8. Remove excess fluid with a tissue or clean kerchief, if required.
9. Wait for at least 5 minutes before applying another drop of same or different medicine.
10. Consult your doctor or pharmacist if burning feeling after application of eye drop lasts more than few minutes.

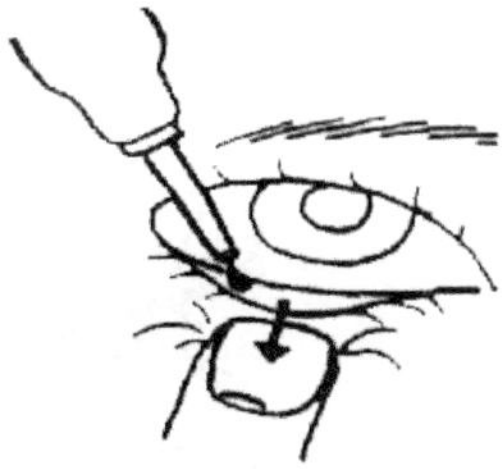

Step 4 and 5 [Source: WHO's Guide to Good Prescribing]

Instruction to parents for children's use:

1. Ask the child to lie back with head straight.
2. Ask the child to close the eyes.
3. Drip the drop into the corner of the eye.
4. Ask the child to keep the head straight.
5. Remove excess fluid.

Eye Ointment: Normally the patient needs the assistance of another person in administering the eye ointment. On application they cause blurred vision and the patient needs to be advised not to get alarmed. It is preferable to use at bed time, if once a day use is prescribed, to avoid visual impairment.

The ointments must be kept clean and every effort must be taken to avoid touching the tip of the tube against the eye or anything else.

Instruction to patients:

1. Wash your hands.
2. Do not touch anything with the tip of the tube.
3. Tilt the head backwards a little.
4. Take the tube in one hand, and pull down the lower eyelid with the other hand, to make a gutter.
5. Bring the tip of the tube as close to the gutter as possible.
6. Apply the amount of ointment as advised by doctor.
7. Close the eye for two minutes.
8. Remove excess ointment with a tissue or clean kerchief.
9. Clean the tip of the tube with a tissue and close with the cap.

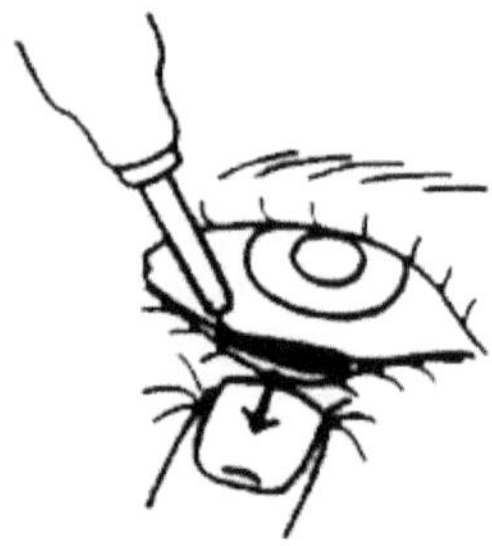

Step 4 and 5 [Source: WHO's Guide to Good Prescribing]

Applicaps: These are soft gelatin capsules containing eye ointment for single application. The capsule is to be pricked with a clean needle or elongated part can be cut with a clean scissor and the contained ointment can be applied as discussed under ointment.

(b) When less is better – Using Eye Drops!

Eyes are the most sensitive organs of our body and the eye drops are most common form of medications used for the treatment of eye disorders. Eye drops directly deliver the desired medication to the eye. Most of the time we believe more is better. Use more than one drop at a time for better therapy. But is not true! Here less is better. Smaller drops are more effective.

The capacity of the eye to retain fluid (eye drop) is limited. A blinking eye can accommodate or retain a volume of maximum 30 μL including the normal tear volume of 7-8 μL. Unblinking eye, on the other hand, can retain only about 10 μL. A single drop of eye drop (solution) delivers around 50 μL which is much higher than the retention capacity eye. Ideally a volume for instilling into eye should be 5-10 μL. The sizable portion of the instilled dose either spills on to the cheek (may cause contact allergy)or is very quickly drained away. Similarly, if multiple drops are applied at time, most of the instilled solution would be lost due to spillage or drainage.

The eye drops are applied to the pocket formed by gently pulling the lower eye lid downward. Upon instillation the lower lid should be released and the eye is kept closed at least for a minute without blinking, rubbing or wiping. The closed eye allows the medication to spread over the eye.

A single drop at a time is advised not only for better therapy but also to minimize waste. This also prevents undesired absorption or contact skin allergy from washed out drops.

In addition to general guidelines for maintaining hygienic practices to maintain sterility of the products, the patients should be educated on the following aspects:

- Only one drop should be used at a time. If second drop is recommended, then allow few minutes before applying next drop.

- If more than one type eye drop is to be applied (different medications), patient should wait at least for three minutes before applying the next drop.
- Wait of at least 15 minutes before putting back the contact lenses.
- Do not use after the expiry date and do not use after 28 days (four weeks) of opening the container.
- Report back to your physicians if the product produces irritation.

CHAPTER 46

Ear Products

Ears are one of the sophisticated organs of the body with impressive engineering feat of construction and operation. Sometimes, like other organs we face the pathologic conditions of ears and it becomes necessary to rectify or correct the problem through the use of medicines. The medicines used in the ear for rectification of its pathologic condition are called 'ear products'. They are also known as otic or aural products.

They are usually simple solutions or suspensions or ointments of medicaments designed to exert a local effect in the ear, to soften wax, to treat local inflammation and infection, or to relive pain. They are available as ear drops and ear ointments.

Ear Drops: They are generally formulated either as solutions or suspensions in a vehicle of anhydrous glycerin or propylene glycol. Water is avoided as it supports microbial growth. They are packed in small glass or plastic containers with a dropper and volume is usually 5-15 ml.

It is desirable to warm the ear drops to body temperature before instillation into the ear. The warmer solution helps improving the degree and rate of drug mixing with cerumen(wax) and thus improving contact of drug with external ear membrane. Beside this, warmer solution provides subjective relief of pain for the patient. The drops are to be warmed holding in hand and heating over a flame or warm water be avoided as they are likely to cause overheating. The patient needs to be explained the way of warming the drops prior to use every time. Suspension drops requires the "Shake Well Before Use" instruction every time.

The ear drop needs to run into deeper on instillations and hence the ear lobe should be held up and back while the ear lobe of child should be held down and back. The number of drops required to be instilled is generally 1 or 2 drops, which the ear canal can easily hold. If too much pressure is used to administer ear drop damage may occur to the tympanic membrane. A cotton pledget may be placed in the ear canal to minimize leakage.

The ear drop in the ear canal is likely to cause some hearing loss or stinging or both because of low pH of the product. The patient needs to be informed of this expected problems so that he/she does not get frightened when experience similar problems while using the ear drops.

The drops are to be used for recommended period of duration and the patients should be asked or advised to use drops for 3 days beyond the time ear symptoms disappear, especially in case of antimicrobials drops.

The ear drop bottle may not be full. The empty space volume is for providing proper drop control.

The necessary administration steps required to be 142ounseled is given below:

1. Wash your hands.
2. Warm the ear drop by keeping them in hand or the armpit for several minutes.
3. Tilt head sideways or lie on one side with ear upward.
4. Apply the amount of drops prescribed.
5. Wait five minutes before turning to the other ear.
6. Use cotton wool to close the ear canal after applying the drops ONLY if the manufacturer explicitly recommends this.
7. Do not rinse dropper after use. Wipe the tip of the dropper with a clean tissue and keep the container tightly closed.
8. Do not touch the applicator tip to any surface including the ear.

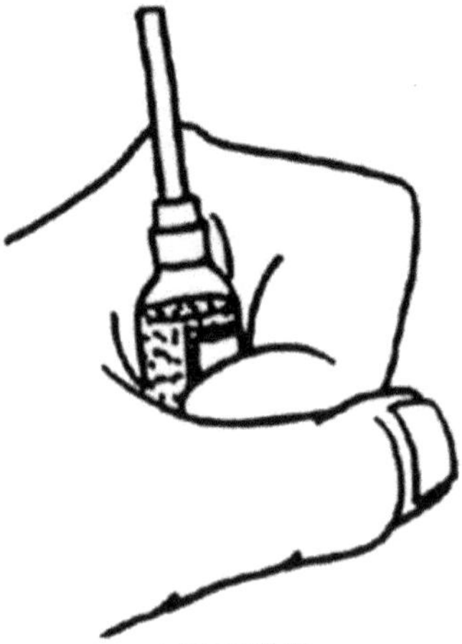

Step - 2

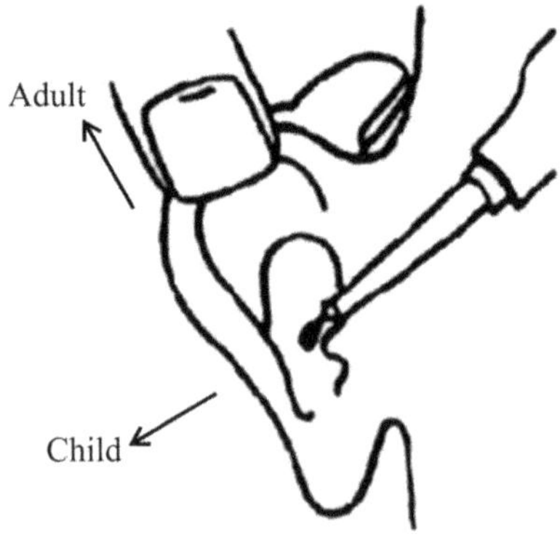

Step - 3 and 4

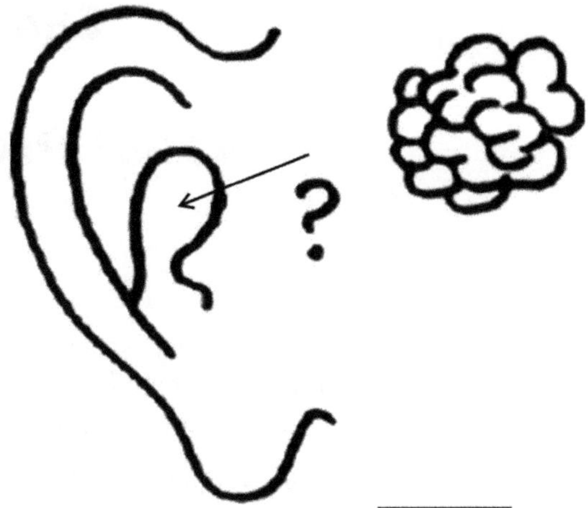

Step - 6

Ointments: As the ointment melts at body temperature, the product should be placed in the ear canal while the patient is lying on his side. Use of cotton pledget is recommended to minimize the unsightly appearance or staining of bed clothing due to leakage.

Like any other medicine, these ear products need to be kept in a safe place away from reach of children. They require to be stored in a dry and cool place. The patient needs to be instructed on these aspects of storage too to improve medicine use and avoid any mishap.

CHAPTER 47

Nasal Products

Nose is the external opening of respiratory system and houses the apparatus for filtration and temperature and humidity control of inspired air. It is the organ of smell and plays a vital role in health maintenance.

In addition to susceptibility to nose injury because of location, the nose is associated with many disorders such as infections, nosebleeds etc. The drugs can be administered directly to the nose as local application or systemically to treat such nose disorders. The local drug delivery offers advantage like less toxicity or side effects as little amount of drug is employed. However, some patients experience the irritant effects associated due to either drug or the vehicle. Frequent and prolonged use of some nasal drops sometimes cause rebound congestion. Systemic route of drug delivery is necessary for long-term treatment.

Nasal Drops: Patient needs to wash his/her hand with soap and water prior to use nasal drops. It is necessary to blow the nose to clear the nostrils. For maximum penetration with drops, a patient requires to lie down on a flat surface, such as bed, hanging the head over the edge, and then tilting the head back as far as possible.

As most the nasal drops are decongestant and many of them cause rebound congestion, the patient should not use the drops longer than prescribed or not beyond 5 days.

The instruction to patient follows:

1. Wash the hand thoroughly.
2. Blow the nose.
3. Sit down and tilt head backward strongly or lie down on a flat surface; keep the head straight.
4. Insert the dropper one centimeter into the nostril.
5. Apply the number of drops as prescribed.
6. Immediately afterward tilt head forward strongly (head between knees).

7. Sit up after a few seconds; drops will then drip into pharynx.
8. Repeat the procedure for the other nostril, if necessary.
9. Rinse the dropper with boiled water.

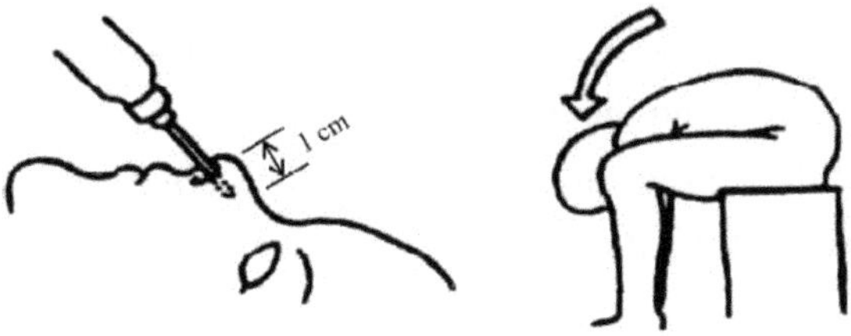

Step 3 and 4

[Source: WHO's Guide to Good Prescribing]

Inhalers: The volatile drug is impregnated to fibrous materials contained in a cylindrical plastic container called inhaler. They are used to treat nasal congestion.

They are effective as long as the volatile drug component remains. The patient needs to be advised to place the inhaler in the nostril and inhale the vapour. To ensure that the drug is not lost during non use, the cap of the inhaler should be tightly closed. The patient should be cautioned that excessive use may cause nasal edema and rebound congestion.

Sprays: These contain solution of medicament(s) and are packed in flexible plastic bottles designed to deliver a fine spray through a small orifice when the bottle is squeezed or may be packed in pressurized container (aerosols). The aerosols will be discussed separately.

Patient should not lie on a flat surface. If this is performed, there is a chance that administration would be enhanced by the prone position. It is better to merely have the patient tilt the head back while standing and gently squeeze the bottle between thumb and forefinger to deliver the medications in a fine spray of mist.

The following are the instruction to patient:

1. Blow the nose.
2. Sit with head tilted forward.
3. Shake the spray.
4. Insert the tip in one nostril.

5. Close the other nostril and mouth.
6. Spray by squeezing the bottle and sniff slowly.
7. Remove the tip from the nose and bend the head forward strongly (head between the knees).
8. Sit up after few seconds; the spray will drip down the pharynx.
9. Breath through the mouth.
10. Repeat the procedure for other nostril, if necessary.
11. Rinse the tip with boiled water.

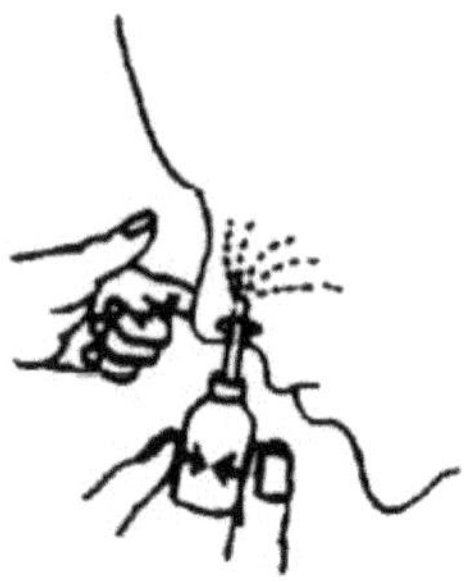

Step 4 and 5

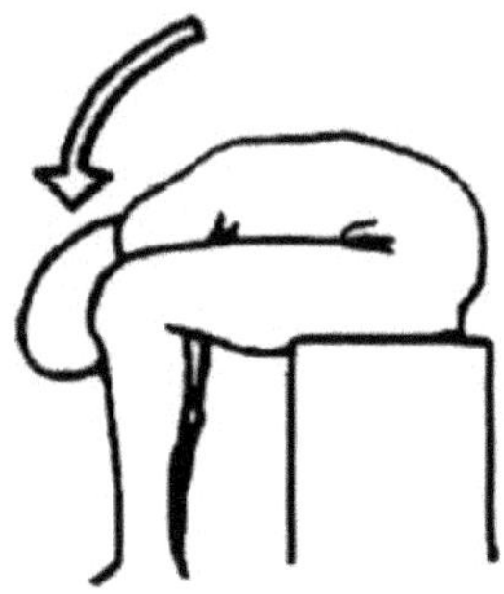

Step 7

[Source: WHO's Guide to Good Prescribing]

CHAPTER 48

Metered Dose Inhalers

Winter is perhaps the worst time for asthmatics. With winter setting in, the asthma patients need to gear themselves with keeping the asthma medications handy. Asthma is a disease of the respiratory system where people have sensitive airways in their lungs. When it happens, the airways become narrow making it hard for them to breathe.

Asthma is increasing in prevalence in our society. It is reported that around 15% of our population suffer from either a mild or severe form of asthma. The burden is believed to be more than 15 million in our country. The common symptoms of asthma are unproductive cough, wheezing (a fine whistling sound), chest tightness and sensation of shortness of breath.

There are three main factors that cause the airways to become narrow: the inside lining of the airways becomes red and swollen (inflammation), extra mucous may be produced, and the muscle around the airways tightens (bronchoconstriction). Asthma attacks are commonly caused by exposure to specific allergens, air pollutants, industrial chemicals, or infection. They can be caused by exercise too especially in cold air. Even the emotional factors can worsen the condition. The allergens usually responsible for asthma attacks are dust mites, pollen, animal fur and feathers. Sudden change of temperature and cold air of winter are known triggers of asthma. This time of the year being the deewali season, people get their homes renovated. Fumes from paints and dusts from carpentry too are problematic. Pollution and smoke produced during cracker bursting and firework display are often dreaded for asthmatic patients. In all such situations, the asthmatics do need to keep their inhalers handy.

The goal of medicine therapy is to control asthma symptoms, to reduce frequency of attacks, and severity of exacerbations, and to reverse air flow obstruction. Basically there are two groups of medicines used in the management of asthma (there are other categories of medicines too):

use of bronchodilators and anti-inflammatory agents. The bronchodilators cause dilation of the airways and the anti-inflammatory agents reduce the inflammation in the airways. When there is little response to bronchodilators, the anti-inflammatory agents like steroids (corticosteroids) are advised to be used to quickly regain control of asthma. The asthma medicines can be: taken orally, by injection or by inhalation. Inhalation is preferred because quick relief can be obtained by this route.

With inhalation medication goes directly to the lungs and smaller doses may be necessary with fewer side effects. There are two types of inhalers: aerosol inhaler (puffer) and dry powder inhaler. The aerosol inhalers are more common. Asthma care depends on the proper use of medication and inhalers. Under treatment and suboptimal therapy are the major factors that contribute to morbidity and mortality.

Learn the use of inhalers to get the maximum benefits.

Aerosol inhalers are pressurized package when pressed it releases one dose. They are also known as metered dose inhalers. Though earlier chlorofluorocarbons were used to build pressure in the inhaler, based on Montreal protocol the present day asthma inhalers are now environment friendly. To get maximum benefit from the use of inhalers, it is necessary that they are properly used. The following guidelines are helpful (most of the inhalers come with user guidelines and the patients need to read and follow):

1. Remove the plastic cap that covers the mouthpiece.
2. Shake the inhaler vigorously before taking each dose.
3. Breathe out as fully as you comfortably can.
4. Tilt the chin up and hold the inhalers upright keeping mouth piece in your mouth. Create a seal with your lips.
5. Breathe in deeply as you press down on the can with your index finger.
6. When you complete breathe in, hold your breath as long as you comfortably can.
7. Remove the inhaler from the mouth and replace the cover.

If you need more than one dose (puff), repeat the process from 2-6 after 1 minute of administering the first dose. If steroid inhaler is used, rinsing mouth after each use is necessary. The whole process requires good coordination between pressing down the canister and breathe in. When the coordination is a problem, inhalers can be used with a spacer device for ensuring more medication reaching lungs.

Like appropriate use of inhalers, it is important to maintain them. The inhalers should be cleaned daily. To do this, remove the can from the plastic case. Rinse the plastic case and cap in warm water preferably under running water. Dry thoroughly and replace the metal can into the case. Put the cap on the mouthpiece. This would keep the mouth piece free of particles and prevent clogging.

Here are few general guidelines for appropriate use of inhalers and proper management of your asthma:

- Do not self medicate. The types of medicines used to treat asthma attacks are quite strong. If used incorrectly, they may have an immediate and dangerous effect on the health of the user.
- Learn to use your inhalers correctly. Discuss with your doctor or pharmacist.
- Do not use more or less than the recommended dose without consulting your doctor.
- Regularly check that your inhaler is not empty.
- The inhalers are pressurized packs. Do not puncture. Do not discard them into fire too.
- Try to avoid the triggering factors that cause asthma or that worsen your asthma.
- If you experience any side effect of the medicine using, report to your doctor or pharmacist.

CHAPTER 49

Rectally Administered Products

The various types of medicines are administered directly to/through rectum. These medicines are suitably made to release the drug as quickly as possible. Usually, when medicines cannot be given orally, this type of administration is preferable to giving injections. The medicines administered through this route provide local action or systemic action.

Though these medicines (rectally administered products) may cause little inconvenience to the patients, they can be self administered. The most common form of the rectally used products is suppositories. The suppositories are solid at room temperature but will melt or dissolve as they are inserted into the rectum.

Here are the instructions for their use:

- Wash your hands.
- Remove the covering (unless too soft). If the suppository is too soft, keep in the fridge to get hardened.
- Moisten the suppository with cold water.
- Lie on your side with lower leg straightened out and upper leg drawn towards the chest.
- Lift the upper buttock, expose the rectal area and insert the suppository with tapered end first.
- Insert at least for about one inch. If not inserted far enough the suppository may get expelled, in such case, reinsert again.
- Hold closed the buttocks after insertion for few seconds. If possible remain quiet for sometimes and in bed for about 15 minutes.
- Wash your hands and try not to have bowel movement during the first hour.

CHAPTER 50

Vaginally Administered Products

Contraception and infection are the main indications for drug or device administration to vagina. A variety of spermicidal products are available for vaginal use. Vaginal infections can also be treated locally. The common forms of these medicines are available as Vaginal tablets, suppositories, creams, ointments and jellies. Often an applicator is necessary for their use. It is necessary to remember even if they are tablets, they are not meant for swallowing. The administration guidelines are:

Vaginal Tablets and Suppositories

- Wash your hands.
- Remove the foil wrapping from the tablet.
- Moisten the tablet by holding it under warm water for few seconds and then place it into the open end of the applicator.[Pull the plunger until it stops. Then keep the tablet in the cup at the end of the barrel where it will fit snugly and remain in place.].
- Lie on your back with knees elevated and slightly apart.
- Gently insert the applicator with the tablet/suppository in front into the vagina as far as possible. Do not use force. This deposits the tablet deep inside the vagina.
- Depress the plunger to release the tablet. Lie down for a few minutes to prevent expulsion.
- Withdraw the applicator and discard if disposable one.
- Clean the applicator with warm or soapy water. Rinse and dry the applicator and plunger and store in a clean place. Do not use boiling water that may soften the applicator.
- Wash your hands.

Douching immediately after medicine administration should be avoided.

Vaginal creams, ointment and gels: They may be administered with or without applicator. The cream should be stored in such condition that it is not cold at the time of insertion. The instruction guidelines are:

- Wash your hands.
- Remove the cap from the tube.
- Attach the applicator to the tube.
- Fill the applicator by squeezing and rolling up the tube from the bottom. For easier filling hold the medication tube above the applicator. The applicator is filled when the plunger is pushed out as far as it will go.
- Remove the applicator from the tube and replace the cap.
- Lie on the back with knees bent and apart.
- Insert the applicator into vagina as far as possible.
- Hold the cylinder and with the other hand push the plunger down (similar to operation described under vaginal tablets) to insert the medicine into the vagina.
- Remove the applicator with the plunger depressed.
- Lie as such for sometime after removal of the applicator.
- Clean the applicator with warm or soapy water. Rinse and dry the applicator and plunger and store in a clean place. Do not use boiling water that may soften the applicator.
- Wash your hands

Douching immediately after medicine administration should be avoided.

PART C
Individual Medicines

CHAPTER 51

Pain and Fever Relieving Medicines

(a) Pain Relievers

Almost every one of us suffers from pain at one or other time. The pain itself is not a disease but a symptom of the underlying cause. Very often the pains are successfully treated with common pain killer medicines, but the persistent and serious pains require medical attention or advice. The pain is also often associated with inflammation. The group of medicines that are used to relieve pain and inflammation are scientifically known as analgesic and anti-inflammatory medicines.

The commonly used pain killer medicines contain one or two of the following medicines: Aspirin, Paracetamol, Ibuprofen, Naproxen, Diclofenac and Piroxicum. Except paracetamol all others have anti-inflammatory action. They are used for treatment of arthritis, muscle ache, dental pain, most surgical pain, fever, headache, menstrual cramps and athletic injury.

Take pain relieving medicines after food to minimise the gastric side effects. Do not take them more than few days without doctor's advice.

Aspirin is the oldest and one of the most inexpensive analgesics and works well to lower fever. It can cause heartburn, indigestion and peptic ulcer as side effects. Buffered aspirin or enteric-coated preparations reduce this problem. The following guidelines are important for using this medicine as analgesic:

- Avoid during pregnancy and children below 12 years.
- Do not take if you are bleeding or before surgery.
- Avoid if you are asthmatic as it may trigger asthma.
- Avoid if you have gastric problem like peptic ulcer.

Paracetamol is one of the safest pain reliving medicines, which can be used during pregnancy and children. It is also fever-reducing medicine. The larger doses for long periods could be serious with liver and kidney damage. People who consume alcoholic drinks are at higher risk of liver damage.

Ibuprofen, Naproxen etc. are very effective in lower doses for muscle and joint pains, inflammation and pain with monthly bleeding. Like aspirin they too can cause gastric problems like indigestion, nausea, heartburn, stomach pain and ulcer. Ibuprofen may trigger asthma in susceptible patients.

- They should not be taken before surgery or people with stomach ulcer.

All these pain-relieving medicines should be used for mild to moderate pain. For moderate to severe or ongoing pain, stronger medicines are available and should be used under medical advice only. They should not be used for self-care for more than 7-10 days. If the pain persists, consultation with the doctor is advisable.

The adherence to following guidelines will promote safe and effective medications of these categories of medicines:

- ✓ Always take these medicines with food or antacid.
- ✓ Swallow with full tumbler of water.
- ✓ Try the weakest pain medicine first and use stronger one only if needed.
- ✓ Treatment for ongoing pain should be given regularly. Don't wait until the pain returns before the next dose.
- ✓ Avoid combinations of these medicinal ingredients unless specially prescribed.
- ✓ Inform or consult the doctor or pharmacist if you are allergic to any of these medicines, have bleeding problem or high blood pressure.
- ✓ If symptoms persist, consult your doctor before further continuing these medicines.

(b) Pain Killers: Pill Poppers – A Word of Caution!

Following night long tooth ache, Ashok went to the neighbourhood friendly pharmacy seeking a quick remedy. The pharmacist gave him few painkiller tablets. Just the previous day, he read an article in newspaper cautioning the use of painkillers as they are associated with several side effects. Ashok is now confused; whether to take them or are there safer alternatives? Yes, it is not the issue of Ashok alone. There are many of us who depend on the painkillers for maintaining routine daily activities.

Most of the painkillers belong to a group called non-steroidal anti-inflammatory drugs (NSAIDs) and are widely used to treat pain and fever from many different long- and short-term medical conditions such as arthritis, menstrual cramps, headaches, colds, and the flu. NSAIDs are available by prescription and over the counter products. The USFDA, the drugs regulatory authority of United States of America, has just issued warning "non-aspirin NSAIDs increase the chance of a heart attack or stroke". There are several medicines in this group, the most common being, ibuprofen, diclofenac, acceclofenac, naproxen, piroxicam, celecoxiband indomethacin. These medicines are usually associated with gastric irritation, discomfort and sometimes gastric bleeding. In order to prevent the side effects, the medicines are advised to be taken after food and often with gastric acid reducing medicines. But the gastric acid reducing medicines are too not free of side effects. Especially the proton pump inhibitors cause serious side effects on continued use.

Ever since the voluntary withdrawal of rofecoxib (Vioxx) from international marketing following several reports of cardiovascular deaths in 2004, there has been a great deal of interest on safety of NSAIDs. The present FDA warning has once again highlighted the potential risk of the pain killers. This will have far reaching consequences on use and marketing of the NSAIDs. They can increase the risk of heart attack or stroke in patients with or without heart disease or risk factors for heart disease. However patients with heart diseases are at higher risk. The risk increases with increasing dose and duration of treatment. The risk of heart attack or stroke can occur as early as the first weeks of using an NSAID. It further warns "Patients treated with NSAIDs following a first heart attack are more likely to die in the first year after the heart attack compared to patients who are not treated with NSAIDs after their first heart attack". USFDA continues advising patients taking NSAIDs should seek medical attention immediately if they experience symptoms such as chest pain, shortness of breath or trouble breathing, weakness in one part or side of their body, or slurred speech.

There is a safer alternative. The topical form of application of NSAIDs is found to be equally effective but much safer. A recent Cochrane review (a good source of evidence based drug therapy) confirmed the effectiveness of topical non-steroidal anti-inflammatory drugs is similar to that of orally administered ones. The study compared the effects of NSAIDs in the form of gel, spray, or cream. Formulations of topical diclofenac, ibuprofen, ketoprofen, piroxicam, and indomethacin demonstrated significantly higher rates of clinical success than matching topical placebo. Gel formulations of diclofenac (as Emugel®), ibuprofen, and ketoprofen, and some diclofenac patches, provided the best effects. The adverse events reported were very minimal. Local skin reactions were mild and transient and similar to placebos. However, topical application is not always feasible.

In spite of NSAIDs' popularity of being clinically effective in relieving pain, they are not free of side effects including potential for causing cardiovascular harms. They can kill the users. "Use NSAIDs at lowest possible dose for shorted possible time" should be the philosophy.

(c) Aspirin: A Common Pain Killer

Aspirin, chemically known as acetyl salicylic acid, is the oldest and least expensive pain killer medicine. It has anti-inflammatory and anti-rheumatic effects and thus has been in use for the treatment of mild to moderate pain. Though it has good temperature lowering effect, it does not correct the cause of fever. The activity of aspirin traces back to its parent compound, salicylic acid. The salicylic acid is too strong to be used as medicine because of its gastric effects like gastric bleeding. Aspirin acts by inhibiting the prostaglandin, the hormone like substances having wide physiological activities.

Prostaglandin protects the digestive tract from the action of stomach acid. Taking aspirin may cause gastrointestinal upset, ulcers or even bleeding. It can also cause heartburn, indigestion and peptic ulcer. The usual adult dose of aspirin is 325 mg to 650 mg orally every 4 to 6 hours. For children recommended dose is 10 to 15 mg per kilogram body weight of the child every 4 to 6 hours. Higher doses are for specific conditions.

Take aspirin after food to reduce gastric side effects.
Do not give to children without doctor's advice.

They are available as tablets only. The liquid preparations are not available because they are not stable. The tablets are available as swallowable type or effervescent type. The swallowable tablets are often enteric coated (mainly used for preventing heart attack). The effervescent tablets (disprin) are meant to be added to a tumbler of water and to be taken while effervescing. The swallowable tablets are to be taken with plenty of water and after food. They must not be taken in empty stomach. The effervescent type preparations and taking after food reduce the risk of gastric damage by this medicine. The enteric -coated tablets are not useful for rapid pain relief.

Aspirin undergoes hydrolysis in presence of moisture. This is manifested by strong odour of vinegar (acetic acid). The tablets must be protected against exposure to moisture. This hydrolysis causes loss of potency.

Aspirin is not recommended for children suffering from influenza or chicken pox. In such situation, the medicine may cause severe reactions such as difficulty in breathing, disorientation etc. (Reye's syndrome). The Reye's syndrome is an acute, potentially fatal illness occurring almost exclusively younger than 15 years. It is preferable not to use aspirin in children and alternative paracetamol may be used. Aspirin use during pregnancy may cause adverse fetal effects, such as low birth weight, increased incidence of haemorrhage in premature infants, still birth, or neonatal deaths. Aspirin's use needs to be avoided during pregnancy, especially in the third trimester.

The general guidelines for safe and effective use of aspirin as pain killer and anti-rheumatic medicine (the use of aspirin in other conditions like preventing cardio vascular events will be discussed separately):

- Use Aspirin for relieving aches and pains of muscles and joints; to lower fever; to relieve symptoms of common cold; to relive pain and fever of rheumatic fever. It is not useful in severe pain such as that result from accident, burns or heart attack or pain in abdomen.
- Take with or after food to reduce gastric side effects. Always swallow with plenty of water.
- Do not use in children without doctor's advice. It can cause serious problems if children have chicken pox or flu like symptoms.
- Inform your doctor or dentist before surgery or dental care that you are taking aspirin. It may cause bleeding problem.
- Be careful. Other medicines like medicines of cough and cold may contain aspirin. There may be additive dose.
- Inform your doctor or pharmacist, if you experience any side or undesirable effects.

(d) Paracetamol: Fever Relieving Medicine

Fever itself is not an illness but a sign of illness. The normal body temperature is around 37°C in healthy persons. A person with temperature higher than 37°C is said to have fever. Most fevers are self-limiting and non-threatening. But it can cause a great deal of discomfort. Some cases it indicates serious underlying pathology, which needs prompt medical attention. Though treatment should target the underlying causes wherever possible, reduction of fever is essential to alleviate discomfort.

Fever is usually caused by infections, often viral. For viral fever, there is no specific anti-infective therapy available. The fever may also be induced by certain medicines or physiologic process or may of unknown origin. Though serious complications of fever are rare, harmful effects like dehydration, convulsion, coma etc., are most likely to occur at temperature above 41°C. It is often a vital sign, which tells how ill the person is, whether he/she is improving, or whether the patient responds to treatment or not. The type of fever often helps in diagnosis.

Paracetamol is one of the most widely used fever reducing medicine, available in variety of brand names. It is also known as acetaminophen. It reduces fever by directly acting on the hypothalamus, heat-regulating centre of the brain. The body heat is reduced by vasodilation and sweating.

Do not take more than 4 g of paracetamol per day to avoid liver toxicity.

When used appropriately, it rarely causes severe toxicity or side effects. Acute poisoning often occurs because of large dose swallowing and is manifested by nausea, vomiting, drowsiness, confusion, liver tenderness, low blood pressure, cardiac arrhythmia, jaundice and acute hepatic and renal failure. Hepatotoxicity (liver toxicity) may result in excessive dose. The minimum toxic dose is around 10 g (140mg/kg body weight). High doses are potentially fatal. Realizing its toxicity, the Government has restricted its content to be of maximum 325 mg in combination medicines. In case of poisoning or experiencing toxicity, consulting a doctor is very much essential. Paracetamol is normally recognized as safe for use during pregnancy.

Paracetamol is available at variety of strength and dosage form. For children they are available as syrup or suspension or dispersible tablets. For adult they are available as tablets. Paracetamol is also available as injections. The adult dose of paracetamol for fever is 500 mg to 1 gram every 4-6 hours, with not exceeding 4 gram daily. Children require lower dosage: 3 months to 1 year: 60-125 mg; 1-5 years: 120-250 mg; 6-12 years: 250-500 mg; these doses may be repeated every 4-6 hours (usually not exceeding 4 doses in 24 hours). The strength of paediatric liquid preparations is often different for different products like 125 mg/5 ml or 250 mg/5 ml. One needs to be careful for dosing.

The tablet(s) are to be swallowed with plenty of water. The suspensions need to be shaken before measuring dose. The dispersible tablets are to be kept with water in a spoon and when dispersion is complete, they need to be swallowed with plenty of water. Swallowing plenty of water along with medicines has beneficial effects. Only linctuses are advised to be swallowed /taken without water.

Paracetamol has pain-relieving activity too. There are other medicines like aspirin and ibuprofen, which can be used for relieving fever. The details on them will be discussed in some other time. Body sponging with tepid water can also be used for heat dissipation to relieve fever. Body sponging usually in children is uncomfortable. Ice water bath or sponging with hydroalcoholic solution is uncomfortable and unnecessary. Wearing light clothing, removing blankets, maintaining room temperature at around 25°C, and drinking plenty of fluids is recommended.

Following are the few tips for safe and effective use of Paracetamol:

- Do not exceed the daily dose of more than 4 gram to avoid liver damage or toxicity.
- Avoid fasting.
- Do not drink alcohol during paracetamol use. It increases the toxicity.
- Be aware of other OTC medicines. Some of the medicines for cough, cold, pain or allergy may contain paracetamol. Check the total dose of paracetamol.
- Do not use in children younger than 2 years without medical advice.

- Do not take paracetamol for more than 3 days for fever unless your doctor advises. If the symptoms persist, worsen, or if new symptoms arise, consult your doctor.
- Consult your doctor before using paracetamol in children with predisposed seizure.

(e) Revisiting Paracetamol!

Paracetamol (often called Acetaminophen) is perhaps one of the most widely used medicines and is believed to be safe. This has been indicated as antipyretic and analgesic; available without prescription and falls under schedule K of the Drugs and Cosmetics Act. Sale of simple paracetamol tablets does not require even a sale license for selling in villages subject to certain restrictions. In addition to simple paracetamol in a product there are many combination products in the market. Following the USFDA guideline the Government of India too issued instruction to restrict the quantity of paracetamol to 325 mg only in a combination product. This is just to avoid liver injury risk. Even after the Government of India's guideline, it has been reported thatmany combination products still continue to have more than 325 mg paracetamol.

Following the discussion on availability of higher amount of paracetamol in Fixed Dose Combinations at Drugs Consultative Meeting, Country's highest regulatory authority, Drugs Controller General India (DCGI), issued clarification that limit of 325 mg Paracetamol is applicable only to FDCs with other pain relieving or anti-inflammatory agents. Other FDCs and single ingredient product can continue to have 500 mg or higher strength. The USFDA's direction issued in 2011 to limit quantity of paracetamol to 325 mg per dose in prescription only medicines is complied by many pharmaceutical companies. Ironically the USFDA has not bothered to issue instruction on Over the Counter Paracetamol products and these products continue to have the strength at 500 mg per dose. The liver injury risk is same whether the paracetamol product comes under prescription only medicine or over the counter one. The liver injury risk is related to the quantum of paracetamol. USFDA statement continues "there is no evidence to show that higher amounts of acetaminophen doses provide additional benefit that outweighs the added risks for liver injury". The study has shown that some adults developed early signs of liver toxicity after taking just 4 grams per day of acetaminophen, or just over eight "extra-strength" tablets of 500 mg acetaminophen in a day. The current recommended daily maximum dose is 3 grams per day, the amount in six 500 mg tablets.

The different strength of products both for paediatric and adult use add further confusion. The patients often fail to recognize the duplication and continue taking two or more products containing paracetamol leading to severe liver injury. Even in absence of USFDA's clear instruction; the Public Citizen Health Research Group, a prestigious civil society group in USA, advises the consumers not to take more than 325 mg paracetamol per dose not exceeding 3 g daily. This makes a sense and same should be applicable to Indian population too! We can at least advise the patient to limit to 6 tablets of paracetamol 500 mg per day and limiting the total amount of paracetamol to not more than 3 g per day from all sources. The patient needs to be advised to avoid alcoholic drinks while taking paracetamol. This is all in the best interest of the patient, a fundamental component of medical ethics.

(f) Nimesulide: a Not to Use Medicine!

The medicine is not licensed for use in countries like United States, Canada, United Kingdom, Australia, New Zealand etc. Even the neighbouring countries Sri Lanka and Bangladesh have not allowed or stopped the marketing in their territory. But this is available freely in our country even for paediatric use. It is nimesulide.

Nimesulide is a non-steroidal anti-inflammatory drug approved for treatment of acute pain, symptomatic treatment of osteoarthritis and primary dysmenorrhoea in adolescents and adults. The drug was first discovered by a US company, but its use was never in America. However, it is in use in several countries across the world. Recently the Irish and Singapore authority have suspended the use of nimesulide. The European Medicine Agency has banned the use of nimesulide in children below 12 years.

Do not use Nimesulide for simple fever. Do not use Nimesulide in children. Its use in children is banned.

Nimesulide has antipyretic activity (fever reducing) and for which it has been widely used in our country including in children. It seems to have hypothermic properties and it brings down temperature even when it is normal. It is available as tablets and suspensions. There are many combination medicines of nimesulide in Indian market and they are reported to be irrational and unscientific.

No medicine is absolutely safe. Every medicine has side effects. But it is the benefit-risk ratio that decides the usefulness of a drug. Nimesulide is associated with high liver toxicity which is often fatal. The European Agency for the Evaluation of Medicinal Products have revaluated the use of nimesulide and confirmed that the benefits outweigh risks. But it asserts the need of restricting the duration of use to ensure that the risk of patients developing liver problem is kept to a minimum. The use of systemic formulations: tablets, suspensions etc., be restricted to 15 days.

Though the use of nimesulide has been under scan by various drug regulating authorities in the world, recently the drug is under focus Pharmacovigilance programme in India. The government is yet to generate data on its adverse effects. In our country we do not have a good documentation system. Till government makes a decision, the public need to protect their health from ill effects of using the hazardous nimesulide. Not only they should restrict its use to adults to the conditions mentioned above but they should also be aware of that this is not safe for use when one has liver, kidney or gastrointestinal bleeding problems. The Government has banned its use in children. The recommended dose is 100 mg twice a day.

Guidelines

- Never use in children. If doctor prescribes, insist on an alternative.
- If used in adult, restricts its use for treatment of acute pain, symptomatic treatment of painful osteoarthritis and primary dysmenorrhoea for systemic action (when tablets are to be swallowed). Symptomatic relief of pain associated with sprains and acute tendonitis (painful joint disorder) for topical use.
- While using for adults, restricts its use for not more than 15 days.
- Do not use in hepatic or liver problem condition, ulceration, or kidney malfunctioning situation.
- It is a prescription only medicine. Do not self medicate with this.
- Keep all medicines out of reach of children.

(g) Non-Steroidal Anti-Inflammatory Drugs (NSAIDs) in Pain Management

The introduction of some COX – 2 (cyclooxygenase isozymes) inhibitors and their subsequent withdrawal from the market brought serious concern on use of pain relieving medicines. The COX – 2 inhibitors like valdecoxib and rofecoxib were instant hits in pain management as they appeared to cause fewer episodes of serious gastro-intestinal toxicity compared to other available Non-Steroidal Anti-Inflammatory Drugs (NSAIDs). Sooner they were found to be more damaging than the other NSAIDs and they were banned or withdrawn from use due to increased cardiac events. Many litigations followed and the pharmaceutical companies were accused of withholding the cardiovascular events data reported during clinical trials.

The NSAIDs are an important group of pain relieving medicines and have been in use for a variety of pain condition though they differ in their effectiveness. They have significant use in patients with arthritis, low-back pain and soft tissue pain. They do differ in their side effects too. Gastrointestinal bleeding and perforations are common and serious adverse events. These serious events lead to hospitalization and even deaths. The factors known to be responsible for this adverse effect are: types and dose of the drug, use of combination, use of other drugs – anticoagulants, steroids, smoking, alcohol use, older age and patient's susceptibility. Patients with history of ulcer are at more risk. The risk of toxicity increases with increasing dose and length of treatment. Aspirin, the common NSAID, is usually available as plain aspirin, enteric coated aspirin and effervescent aspirin. Though initially it was believed that enteric coated form has less risk than the other two forms, the new evidence suggests that all three forms have equal risk in producing gastric bleeding.

The patients need to be made aware of the risk involved; to stop the use of medicine and report back immediately. Some of the warning signs are: severe abdominal and stomach pain, cramping or burning; severe and continuing nausea, heart burn, indigestion; blood or black, tarry stools; vomiting blood or material that looks like coffee grounds; and spitting blood. This would help preventing major harm to patients.

The recent study reports give a new warning. The use of NSAIDs except naproxen is associated with increased risk of cardiovascular death, fatal and non-fatal myocardial infarction and stroke. The mechanism of this risk factor is related to their effect on COX – 1 and Cox – 2 inhibitors. Diclofenac is found to be completely inhibiting COX – 2 and partially COX – 1 and has the maximum risk of cardiovascular events. On the other hand, naproxen inhibits both COX 1 and COX 2 and has the least cardio vascular risk. The NSAIDs that inhibit COX-2 without complete inhibition of COX-1 has the greatest risk.

All the NSAIDs have almost similar effectiveness. While it is important to make a balance on efficacy and safety in use of medicine, the following few tips would help minimising the harm but providing maximum benefits in pain management:

- Use at the lowest effective dose for the lowest possible time;
- Identify the NSAID with lowest risk profile;
- Exercise caution while selecting diclofenac as it has maximum cardiovascular risk;
- Consider the risk of gastrointestinal bleeding and cardiovascular events before recommending or using.

(h) Topical Pain Killers

"A medical examiner in USA blamed a 17 year old track star's death on the use of too much muscle cream, the kind used to soothe aching legs after exercise". This has been recently reported in a newspaper with a heading, "pain relieving cream kill teen athlete". Though apparently it looks the externally used products are safe, it is not so. It too can cause problem though rarely serious like the reported case, if not properly used. In the reported case, the athlete used too much of methyl salicylate cream causing high level of methyl salicylate in the blood. Abnormal amount of methyl salicylate was absorbed through the skin.

Skeletal muscle pain is common and caused by sprain and strain and cramps. Sprain is a partial or complete rupture of ligament. Strain is a partial tear of muscles and cramp is painful spasmodic contraction of a muscle. The strenuous exercise often causes these problems. The sprains and strains are difficult to distinguish as they have common symptoms like pain, swelling, bruising, loss of some functions and gradual stiffening. However sprains occur at joints. When these injuries occur, the muscles become sore and painful and movements become difficult. Muscle cramps (spasms) can occur in any skeletal muscle.

Cramps are usually harmless and do not need to be treated. Stretching and massaging the affected area followed by rest or reduced activity will loosen muscle. But stretching should be done carefully to avoid muscle strain. For persistent cramps, application of warm wet compress, heating pad or hot water bottle provides relief. They can usually be prevented by avoiding exercise after eating and stretching the muscles before exercise and sleeping.

Self treatment of sprains and strains are intended to get relief from pain and swelling, restore functions of the affected areas and prevent further injury. However, serious cases require immediate medical attention. In addition to rest, application of ice, use of elastic bandage, some external analgesics are extremely useful. In this article, a group of medicines called counter irritants are only discussed. These topical counter irritants are applied to the intact skin to decreasing the pain and discomfort associated with minor aches and pains of muscles and joints.

They usually offer good relief for several hours but they should be used correctly to maximise benefits with little or no risks.

Counter irritation is the paradoxical pain relieving effect achieved by producing less severe pain to counter a more intense one. When these counter irritants are applied to the skin at pain sites, they produce a mild, local and inflammatory reaction, which provide relief at another site that is usually adjacent to, or underlying, the skin surface being treated. The intensity of response depends on the irritant concentration and duration of contact with the skin. The degree of irritation must be controlled; otherwise strong irritation may cause allergic reactions such as erythema and blistering.

Avoid contact with eyes and mucous membranes.
Do not apply to broken skin.

Commonly used counter irritant analgesic products have one or some of the following ingredients: allyl isothiocyanate, methyl salicylate, turpentine oil, camphor, menthol, histamine dihydrochloride, methyl nicotinate, capsicum, capsicum oleoresin, and capsaicin. The products are available as liniments, gels, lotions, ointments and sprays. Greaseless and water soluble preparations are cosmetically more acceptable or preferred. Sprays have advantage that they can be sprayed or applied over the affected area without touching either the product or the body part. However, they are costlier. Use of heating pads, excessive after application of methyl salicylate containing product may increase percutaneous absorption (entry into blood through the skin). The systemic availability may increase to a level leading to adverse systemic reactions. This is perhaps the situation of the athlete died after using methyl salicylate sports cream.

Here are few general guidelines for safe and effective use of counter irritant pain killer products:

- While using one must take care to avoid contact with eyes or mucous membranes. Wash your hands after handling these products and before touching eyes or mucous membranes.
- Do not use over abraded, sun burned or damaged skin.
- Do not put a tight bandage or dressing over an area treated with counter irritant product.
- Apply about 3 to 4 times a day and only up to around one week.

- If symptoms persist even after one week of treatment, consult your doctor.
- Do not use these products if you are under treatment with anticoagulants especially warfarin.
- Consult your doctor or pharmacist, if you experience side effects: excessive redness, blistering, vomiting etc.
- Do not use heating pads or other heating devices after application of these products.
- Do not apply after strenuous exercise, especially during hot and humid weather. Apply these products once the body is cooled down.
- Do not use in children below 2 years unless advised by your doctor.
- Keep them out of reach of children.

Topical NSAIDs for acute pain in adults

A recent Cochrane review confirmed the effectiveness of topical non-steroidal anti-inflammatory drugs (NSAIDs) is similar to that of orally administered ones. The study compared the effects of NSAIDs in the form of gel, spray, or cream. Formulations of topical diclofenac, ibuprofen, ketoprofen, piroxicam, and indomethacin demonstrated significantly higher rates of clinical success than matching topical placebo. Benzydamine did not. Gel formulations of diclofenac (as Emugel®), ibuprofen, and ketoprofen, and some diclofenac patches, provided the best effects. The adverse events reported were very minimal. Local skin reactions were mild and transient and similar to placebos.

CHAPTER 52

Gastric Acid Relieving Medicines

(a) Gastric Antacids

Heartburn, indigestion and sour stomach are common problems of many of us. The basic aim of treatment of such problems is to prevent the production of stomach acid or to neutralize the excess acid. Hydrochloric acid is stomach acid. The medicines that are used to reduce acid production should be used only under medical advice. They are prescription only medicines. The acid neutralizing medicines are known as gastric antacids and are over the counter medicines. They are available without prescription. Though they do not completely neutralize the hydrochloric acid in the stomach, they significantly relieve the symptoms for most people by neutralizing almost 99% of acid.

Most of these antacid products are available either in solid or liquid form and contain one or more of the following medicinal ingredients: Sodium Bicarbonate, Magnesium Oxide or Hydroxide, Calcium Carbonate, Magnesium Trisilicate or Carbonate, Aluminium Hydroxide.

Sodium Hydroxide has fast acid neutralizing activity and has been used for decades as kitchen medicine (baking soda). It is an excellent short-term solution but too much use can cause disturbance in acid-base balance of the body. High sodium content may cause problems for people with high blood pressure and such people should avoid this. It can release enough carbon dioxide in the stomach to cause discomfort and belching.

Ideally the combinations of the ingredients described above make good antacids and they are popular too. Antacids with both aluminium and magnesium are found to be quick acting and providing long lasting relief. The side effects of these ingredients are balanced too in the combination. The risk of producing loose motion of magnesium salt is balanced by the constipating effect of aluminium.

Though these antacids are available for self-care without prescription and reasonably safe for use without medical advice, they interact with many prescription medicines, reducing their effects.

Liquid medicines are fast acting than tablets.

Anyone who has heart trouble, high blood pressure or kidney problem should consult doctor before selecting antacids for self care.

For intermittent use, liquids or powders are more efficient than tablets. The tablets are usually chewable types, which are to be crushed by chewing before swallowing. The liquids are suspensions and the bottle is required to well shaken before measuring each dose.

The gas formation is frequently associated with the problems like acidity, heartburn and indigestion. This is usually reflected as excessive belching, abdominal discomfort or cramping, bloating and/or flatulence. Most of the popular brands of antacids contain 'semithicone (MPS)', a defoaming agent to relieve gas. Find below the general guidelines for using antacids more effectively and rationally:

- ✓ Chew antacid tablets thoroughly and follow with a tumbler full of water.
- ✓ Liquid medicines are stronger than tablets. Take tablets during the day at work and liquids at night. Tablets are convenient to carry and use outside home.
- ✓ Take them at least 2 hours apart from other medicines – before or after. The effect of other medicines may get interfered if taken together.
- ✓ Do not take these medications for longer than around 2 weeks without medical advice.

(b) Ranitidine

If the heart burn or excess acidity in the stomach cannot be successfully treated with common gastric antacids, you are often prescribed ranitidine. Ranitidine is a prescription medicine and one requires prescription to buy this from pharmacy. This belongs to Histamin 2 blockers and blocks the release of stomach acid. It is recommended for use to treat ulcers and excess acid in the stomach.

The stomach acid (hydrochloric acid) is secreted to aid digestion. The sphincter at the junction between the esophagus and the stomach prevents these acidic stomach contents from backing up into the esophagus. The esophagus is not designed to tolerate such strong acids. When the reflux occurs, it causes irritation of the esophagus showing the symptoms of chest pain or discomfort (often called heart burn). The problem is more appreciated after meals, when the stomach is full, and when lying down, because gravity no longer keeps the stomach contents in place. The typical bacterial infection together with hyper acidity or the use of many anti-inflammatory medicines causes gastric ulcer. This medicine is very helpful in such situations.

Like other medicines, this ranitidine is also associated with several adverse effects. The most common being the confusion. The elderly persons are at greater risk of this complication. There are some other medicines of this category. These include cimetidine, famotidine, and nizatidine. The medicine should be used with care during liver or kidney problem. Dosage adjustment may be necessary.

Take with doctor's advice only. Do not take for long time.

Ranitidine is available as tablets or injections. The tablets are available at 150 mg and 300 mg strength. The usual dose is 150 mg twice daily or 300 mg once daily.

Follow these guidelines for safe and effective use of this medicine:

- Take this medicine with your doctor's advice and continue for the full course. Do not stop in between as it may cause relapsing of symptoms.

- Take the medicine at the same time of the day: if 2 doses: one at morning and the other at night; if only 1 dose, take only at bed time.
- If you miss the dose: take it as soon as you remember. If it is time for next dose. Skip off the dose, Do not double the dose.
- Tell your doctor before taking the medicines like aspirin, ibuprofen, diclofenac and other pain killers. They may aggravate the ulcers.
- If you experience any of these symptoms, consult your doctor immediately: abdominal pain, chest and back pain, faintness or weakness that is sudden, fever, heartbeat irregular or fast, joint pain, muscle ache, throat sore, tiredness or weakness that is unusual, vision changes, vomiting, wheezing or troubled breathing.

(c) Omeprazole

The Food and Drug Administration of USA has recently cleared Omeprazole that there is no increased risk of heart problems associated with its long term use. This has been in use either alone or in combination with other medicines for treating heart burn and gastric ulcers.

Often we experience the backward travel of liquids and foods from stomach to the oesophagus (a tube from mouth to the stomach). These acidic contents irritate and injure the oesophagus and cause heart burn. The condition is called Gastro-oesophageal reflux disease (GORD or GERD based on spelling of oesophagus).The common symptoms of GORD/GERD are heart burn (burning sensation in the chest which is usually increased by bending, stooping, lying down, or eating), belching, regurgitation of food, nausea and vomiting, vomiting of blood, hoarseness, sore throat, difficulty in swallowing etc. The problem is typically worse after meals, when the stomach is full and when lying down, because gravity no longer keeps the stomach contents in place.

Some of the general measures help in relieving the symptoms that include reduction in weight, avoiding lying down after meals, sleeping with head of bed elevated, taking medications with plenty of water, avoiding dietary fat, caffeine, chocolate etc., and avoiding tobacco.

Take with doctor's advice only. Do not take for long time.

Omeprazole belongs to the family of medicines called proton pump inhibitors. This group of medicines inhibit secretion of stomach acids. Omeprazole is usually available at three strengths: 10 mg, 20 mg and 40 mg capsules. The capsule contains enteric coated granule formulations of Omeprazole. The delayed release capsules are advised for once a day before meals. Omeprazole gets degraded in stomach acids and hence supplied as enteric coated products. Such capsules or tablets are meant for swallowing intact. They are not to be broken, opened, chewed or crushed but to be swallowed whole with plenty of water. Of late Omeprazole is also made available as ordinary capsules (not enteric coated contents) and powders for suspension. Both these preparations contain sodium bicarbonate (baking soda) which decreases the stomach acids so that the Omeprazole does not get degraded. There are some other medicines too in the Proton Pump Inhibitors group: esomeprazole, lansoprazole, pentoprazole, rabeprazole. This group of medicines are reported to cause dependence (habit forming).

If powder is advised, it should be mixed with water before use. The powder is to be mixed with little water (around 15 to 30 ml) and then drink. The contents should be further mixed with water and drink to ensure all medicines are swallowed. In some countries, Omeprazole is available as non prescription medicine. In our country it is prescription only medicine which signifies to be used only on prescription of doctors. It does not give immediate relief of heart burn symptoms and takes about 1-4 days to feel the full benefit. A one month treatment is normally enough to clear up the symptoms.

Though Omeprazole is well tolerated, it often causes side effects which include stomach pain, diarrhoea, constipation, dizziness, cough and back pain. Some of the side effects could be serious. If one experiences rash, hives, itching, swelling of face, throat etc., difficulty breathing or swallowing, hoarseness, muscle spasm, cramping, burning of or tingling of the lips, tongue, hands etc., should consult back the doctor immediately.

Some of the medicines either get affected by Omeprazole or Omeprazole gets affected by them. One must inform doctor that he or she is taking ampicillin (antibiotic), warfarin (anticoagulant), diazepam (minor tranquilizer), digoxin (heart medicine), ketoconazole (anti-fungal), disulfiram (treatment in alcoholism), sleeping tablets, vitamins, iron preparations etc. The doctor may change the dose or monitor the patients carefully.

The guidelines for safe and effective use of Omeprazole in the treatment of GORD:

- Take the medicine as advised on the label of the medicine. Do not crush, open, split, and chew the enteric coated capsules or tablets. Swallow them whole with plenty of water but not with other liquids. Most of these products are taken before meals.
- Maintain the dose as advised by your doctor. Do not take more or less of it or take it more often or for longer period of time.

- If you miss a dose, take the missed dose as soon as you remember. But if it is time for the nest dose, skip off the missed dose and continue with usual schedule. Do not double the dose.
- If you are taking any other medicines including vitamins, you must inform your doctor.
- If you experience any side effects or other unusual experience, consult back your doctor.
- Keep the medication in original package and out of reach of children.

(d) Peptic Ulcer Healing Medicines

Many people suffer from ulcers, sores or holes in the lining of the stomach or the first part of small intestine. These are called peptic ulcers and based on the anatomical positions; they are called either as gastric ulcers (in the stomach) or duodenal ulcers (in the duodenum). Earlier it was believed that spicy food and stress which cause excess acid secretion in the stomach is the root cause of ulcers. But the new research findings confirmed that majority of these ulcers are caused by infection with *Helicobacter pylori* (bacteria). If the test (urea breath test) confirms the presence of *H. Pylori* infection, the eradication of the infection is a part of treatment process. The certain pain killer type medicines like aspirin, ibuprofen, indomethacin etc., too can cause ulceration and are called drug induced ulcers.

Gastric and duodenal ulcers are healed by 4-8 weeks treatment with ranitidine type medicines (H_2 blockers) but there is a chance of relapse requiring maintenance treatment. Relapse can be prevented very successfully by eradicating *H. Pylori* infection. The following regimen is recommended as first line therapy: omeprazole 40 mg daily for 1 week + metronidazole 400 mg three times daily for 1 week + amoxicillin 500 mg three times daily for 1 week. This regimen is based on assumption that the antibiotics are effective. In case of resistance pattern, the doctors may prescribe different regimen.

Complete the course of medicines.

The following are the guidelines for the safe and effective use

- Take the medicines for the prescribed period. Do not stop without consulting your doctor. Not taking properly may lead to resistance.
- If you miss a dose, take the missed dose as soon as you remember. But if it is time for the nest dose, skip off the missed dose and continue with usual schedule. Do not double the dose.

- Promptly report if you experience diarrhoea (amoxicillin may cause), or other side effects or other unusual experience.
- Amoxicillin may reduce the effect of oral birth control pills. Use condoms during this period.
- Take metronidazole with meals to reduce gastric effects.
- Avoid alcohol and smoking during the treatment period. Metronidazole may cause very unpleasant feeling with alcohol.
- Keep the medication in original package and out of reach of children.

Regimens for *Helicobacter pylori*

[The Medical Letter, Vol. 59 (1525), July 17, 2017]

The development of resistance to antibiotics necessitated the need of update treatment protocol. The preferred regimens for *H. pylori* infection are:

	Usual Dosage	Duration	Remarks
Bismuth Quadruple Therapy			
Bismuth subsalicylate	262 or 525 mg qid	10-14 days	First line choice as empiric therapy. This therapy is more effective than triple therapy.
Metronidazole	250 mg qid or 500 mg tid		
Tetracycline	500 mg qid		
a PPI	*		
Concomitant Quadruple Therapy			
Clarithromycin	500 mg bid	10-14 days	The therapy is more effective than triple regimen therapy. It is recommended as first line treatment.
Amoxicillin	1 g bid		
Metronidazole	500 mg bid		
a PPI	*		
Triple Therapy			
Clarithromycin	500 mg bid	14 days	Due to clarithromycin resistance, the regimen becomes less effective. Hence, the regiment is preferred if there is no
Amoxicillin	1 g bid		
a PPI	*		
OR			
Clarithromycin	500 mg bid	14 days	

Contd....

<table>
<tr><td>Metronidazole</td><td>500 mg tid</td><td rowspan="2"></td><td rowspan="2">issue of clarithromycin resistance or when the patient has not been exposed to macrolide antibiotics before for any reason.</td></tr>
<tr><td>a PPI</td><td>*</td></tr>
<tr><td colspan="4">* Proton Pump Inhibitors (PPI):
• Esomeprazole – 20 mg bid or 40 mg once a day
• Lansoprazole – 30 mg bid
• Omeprazole – 20 mg bid
• Pantoprazole – 40 mg bid
• Rabeprazole – 20 mg bid
PPI duration may be longer to heal the ulcer.</td></tr>
</table>

(e) Proton Pump Inhibitors (PPIs) – Hazardous Group of Medicines

The recent US FDA's instruction to write warning on the label of all Proton Pump Inhibitors about 'increased risk of fracture on long term use' is an eye opening for all concerned with medicine use. These groups of medicines are often considered harmless by physicians, pharmacists and the patients as well. They are perhaps one of the most over used drugs category unmindful of risks involved.

As the name implies, the PPIs block the hydrogen-potassium adenosine triphosphatasesystem (proton pump) of gastric parietal cells and inhibit gastric acid secretion. The PPIs are indicated for the treatment of gastric ulcers, gastro-esophageal reflux disease (GERD) with severe symptoms and prevention of upper gastrointestinal bleeding commonly associated with NSAIDs. Unfortunately, they are even used as first choice for mild cases of heartburn (GERD). The available PPIs in the market are: Omeprazole, Lansprazole, Dexlansoprazole, Esmoprazole, Pantoprazole, Rabeprazole and Llaprazole. Esmoprazole is functionally no different from Omeprazole and so as Dexlansoprazole and Lansprazole. But they have significant difference in prices.

> Being hazardous PPIs should be used carefully especially in the common heartburn. Diet, life style changes, and use of safer and cheaper gastric antacids and H_2 blockers are recommended as alternative to PPIs in GERD.

The studies have shown several risks associated with the use of PPIs: modest increase in hip, spine and wrist fracture; dependence on PPIs (rebound acid hyper secretion risk even after four weeks of use); infection risk (*Clostridium difficile* caused diarrhoea and community acquired pneumonia); and Magnesium deficiency risk. The acid secretion in the stomach is based on a delicate hormonal balance gastrin and somatostatin. Any disruption on this balance and consequent normal physiology, as caused by PPIs, would have long term complications. The inhibition of gastric acid secretion might interfere with absorption of calcium and interference with activity of osteoclasts, which could lead to a decrease in bone resorption. This is the possible hypothesis of increased risk of fracture. After use of one month of PPIs, upon withdrawal there is a rebound hypersecretion of acid, requiring higher doses and in consequences acid secretion would not be controlled by PPIs causing long term dependence. The presence of normal quantity of gastric acid acts as barrier for bacteria. The bacteria that get entry are killed by the acidity of the stomach. *Clostridium difficile* infection (CDI) commonly seen in hospitals causing diarrhoea is strongly associated with use of PPIs. H_2 Blockers do not disturb gastric secretion as do PPIs and do not allow CDI. The PPIs induce bacterial over growth (less acidity in the stomach) in upper gastrointestinal tract and these infected secretions when aspirated especially by elderly people leads to pneumonia.

Though there are unquestionable utility of PPIs when indicated, being hazardous they should be used carefully especially in the common heartburn. Diet, life style changes, and use of safer and cheaper gastric antacids and H_2 blockers are recommended as alternative to PPIs in GERD. Eating smaller meals, not lying down for at least three hours after eating, reducing weight if desirable and avoiding alcohol are known strategies that help the GERD patients. Even when PPIs are recommended they should not be given for long term use.

Proton Pump Inhibitors' Use Linked to Kidney Disease:

A recent research report published in prestigious JAMA *Internal Medicine*cautioned that the proton pump inhibitors (PPIs) appear to significantly elevate the chances of developing chronic kidney disease. Earlier it has already been reported that the use of these drugs increase the risk of variety of problems including bone fractures, infections and possibly even heart problems. The PPIs are popular medicines for heartburn, indigestion and acid reflux. Health professionals and the consumers are advised to use them only when needed.

(f) Choice of Proton Pump Inhibitors

The Proton Pump Inhibitors (PPIs) are useful in relieving symptoms of gastroesophageal reflux disease (GERD) and in healing erosive esophagitis and peptic ulcers. The low dose is generally used for initial treatment of GERD. Higher or more frequent dosing may be necessary for treatment of erosive esophagitis, peptic ulcer disease, Zollinger – Ellison syndrome and *Helicobacter pylori* infection.

<table>
<tr><th>Drug</th><th>Dosage Form</th><th>Dose (Adult)</th><th>Instruction to the patient</th></tr>
<tr><td>Esomeprazole</td><td>Oral powder, capsule, tablet, powder for injection</td><td>20 – 40 mg once a day</td><td rowspan="5">The delayed release, sustained release, and enteric coated tablets / capsules are to be swallowed intact without breaking, chewing.

Look at the label to know the type of the product.</td></tr>
<tr><td>Lansoprazole</td><td>Powder for suspension, tablet, capsule</td><td>15 – 30 mg once a day</td></tr>
<tr><td>Omeprazole</td><td>Powder for suspension, tablet, capsule</td><td>20 – 40 mg once a day</td></tr>
<tr><td>Pantoprazole</td><td>Powder, tablet, powder for injection</td><td>40 mg once a day</td></tr>
<tr><td>Rabeprazole</td><td>Capsule, tablet</td><td>20 mg once a day</td></tr>
</table>

All PPIs have similar effectiveness and are well tolerated. Omeprazole and esomeprazole can increase the serum concentration of diazepam and phenytoin. They inhibit the conversion of Clopidogrel to its active form. It is preferable to avoid these combinations. Price or total cost of treatment should be the criteria for preferring PPI.

The PPIs use is associated with increase in hip, spine and wrist fracture; dependence on PPIs (rebound acid hyper secretion risk even after four weeks of use); infection risk (*Clostridium difficile* caused diarrhoea and community acquired pneumonia); and Magnesium deficiency risk. One needs to avoid self-medication and long term use unless doctor advises.

CHAPTER 53

Antibiotics

(a) Antibiotics - Save them for Tomorrow

The discovery of penicillin by Sir Alexander Fleming in 1929 has revolutionized the fight against infections. This was widely used in post world war II infectious patients. This is the first antibiotic. Subsequently many other antibiotics (including other anti-bacterials produced synthetically) are developed. Unfortunately, many of them are becoming useless gradually because of their misuse and over use by us at various levels.

The antibiotics are important categories of medicines used in the prevention and treatment of bacterial diseases. They have been used as a major tool to control bacteria related morbidity and mortality. They are classified based on their strength: bactericidal and bacteriostatic. Bactericidal antibiotics kill bacteria while bacteriostatic antibiotics merely prevent bacteria from multiplying, allowing the body to eliminate the remaining bacteria. In severe infections the bactericidals are more effective.

The different antibiotics work in different ways against specific infections. Like other medicines they too have toxicity. But some are far more dangerous than others. Great care must be taken in selection and use of these categories of medicines. The common antibiotics (including other anti-bacterials): penicillin, ampicillin, amoxicillin, cephalosporins (ceftazidime, ceftriaxone), chloramphenicol, quinolones (ciprofloxacin, norfloxacin), tetracycline, doxycycline, erythromycin, roxythromycin, azithramycin, streptomycin, sulpha drugs, metronidazole, gentamycin etc.

Your doctor decides which antibiotics you do need based on his guessing of infecting organism. When in doubt or when the antibiotics do not work, the doctor advises for isolating the infecting organism and testing its sensitivity. The test result helps the doctor selecting the ideal antibiotic for your problem or infection. Of course, it takes one or two days to get the sensitivity result from microbiological laboratory.

The indiscriminate and improper use of antibiotics results in survival of the fittest selection process for bacteria, which can both inherit and acquire resistance to medicines. Infections treated with wrong antibiotics or far too short time (often in less dose) results in most bacteria being killed while the resistant ones survive to multiply. The misuse and abuse of antibiotics have resulted in development of resistance. This not only threatens health and life but even kill our friendly bacteria located in different parts of the body. The bacterial resistance is a public health hazard, a global threat. The treatment of tuberculosis becomes a challenge now because of this resistance.

If we don't use antibiotics rationally, we contribute to the development of resistance. Use appropriately and only when necessary.

The development of new antibiotics becomes a necessity in the light of resistance problem, but development of new medicines is costly and time consuming with high rate of failure. The only way out to continue our fight against the bacteria (including other microbes) is to prevent the development of resistance so that the existing medicines can be useful for long time. Here are few guidelines for consumers to follow in an effort to use them rationally:

- Do not self medicate. Unfortunately they are available without prescription. They prescription only medicines.
- Do not insist on antibiotics on your visit to doctors or hospitals. Doctor would prescribe if you do need. They should not be taken like vitamins. Follow the dose, frequency and period schedule completely. Even if you feel better mid way, continue the full course as suggested by your doctor.
- Use only recommended dose – not more and not less. Dose depends on the severity of infection and age and weight.
- Avoid them in conditions like common cold. This is a viral infection and does not require antibiotics, but often people use ignorantly troubling their body and wasting their money.

If antibiotics are to continue to save lives, do not use them indiscriminately (use only when needed) and save them for situations when they would be most required.

(b) Penicillin Group of Antibiotics

The discovery of penicillin by Fleming and its subsequent successful use during Second World War brought the penicillin into the regular clinical practice as a powerful weapon against the infectious diseases. Though several antibiotics have been developed later, there has been development of resistance due to indiscriminate use; the penicillin group of antibiotics continue to be useful and important tools against many bacterial infections. They are useful in bacterial infections and are of no value in viral conditions like cough and colds.

The dosages of antibiotics are very important. The correct dose kills bacteria. The fewer doses would not only be ineffective, it would increase the chances of development of resistance. The excess doses are unnecessary and are waste of money. The excess dose may even lead to toxic effects. Though penicillin group of antibiotics are safe to most people, certain persons develop allergic reactions like itching, raised spots or rashes. Often these reactions appear after hours or days after taking these medicines. In few persons (rarely), penicillin causes a dangerous reaction, called allergic shock or anaphylactic shock. This is life threatening. Hence, penicillin should not be used without doctors' advice and without testing for hypersensitivity or allergy. The symptoms of the allergic shock include getting pale, difficulty in breathing and state of shock on injection or swallowing of penicillin.

A person, who has once had allergy to penicillin, should not take any penicillin group of antibiotics. The next time the reactions would be worse and often life threatening. Injectable penicillin is usually reserved for severe and dangerous infections. Oral penicillin is enough for most infections. The oral penicillin is effective or useful in abscessed or infected teeth, widespread impetigo, ear infection, sinusitis, sore throat, some skin infections etc.

Complete the course of medicine.
Adhere to medication schedule.

Phenoxymethylpenicillin (Penicillin V): This is available as tablet as well as dry powder for oral suspension. The usual dose for infections caused by sensitive bacteria is 500 mg every 6 hours. But dose can be increased in severe infections.

- Always take penicillin on empty stomach (one hour after or two hour before meals).
- Take the entire course of medicine prescribed even if you feel better.
- Report the experience of unusual rash, fever or chills to your doctor or pharmacist.
- Use this medicine only on medical advice.

Ampicillin and Amoxicillin are wider range penicillins. These broad spectrum antibiotics are safer than other broad spectrum antibiotics. They are useful even in children and babies. They are interchangeable as they have similar activities but they differ in doses. They are used to treat wide range of infections including ear infections, respiratory tract infections, urinary tract infection, dental abscess, gonorrhoea etc. Amoxicillin is preferred over ampicillin especially in ear infection, respiratory tract infection and urinary tract infection. Amoxicillin causes less diarrhoea than ampicillin.

Amoxicillin is sometimes combined with Clavulanic acid to widen the spectrum of bacterial activity and becomes useful against amoxicillin – resistant bacteria. The general guidelines for safe and effective use:

Amoxicillin (available as capsules or oral powders for making as syrup):

- The usual adult dose is 500 mg three times a day.
- Do not take, if you are allergic to penicillin.
- Do not miss the dose. Take at evenly spaced times to keep a constant level of drug in body fluids. If it is time for next dose, skip the missed dose. Do not double the dose.
- Report immediately if you experience diarrhoea.
- Stop taking this medicine and get emergency help if you experience difficulty in breathing, light headedness, skin rash, hives, itching or wheezing.
- Complete the full course of the medicine even if you feel better.
- Take the medicine on medical advice only.

Ampicillin (available as capsule or oral powders for syrup or injection):

- The usual adult dose is 500 mg four times a day.
- Do not take, if you are allergic to penicillin.
- Do not miss the dose. Take at evenly spaced times to keep a constant level of drug in body fluids. If it is time for next dose, skip the missed dose. Do not double the dose.
- Report immediately if you experience diarrhoea.
- Stop taking this medicine and get emergency help if you experience difficulty in breathing, light headedness, skin rash, hives, itching or wheezing.
- Complete the full course of the medicine even if you feel better.
- Take the medicine on medical advice only.

(c) Macrolide (Erythromycin) Group Antibiotics

Erythromycin group of antibiotics (macrolides) have similar spectrum of activities as that of penicillin group. These medicines are used as an alternative in penicillin allergic patients for the treatment of respiratory infections, whooping cough, legionnaires' disease and campylobacter enteritis. They are more expensive than penicillins.

Erythromycin: Erythromycin is available as tablets, enteric coated tablets, and powder for infusion (slow injection) and also in other forms. The enteric coated tablets are to be taken as they are. They must not be broken. The usual dose is 250-500 mg every 6 hours (four times daily). The common adverse effects are nausea, vomiting, abdominal discomfort; urticaria, rashes and other allergic reactions; reversible hearing loss after large doses etc.; erythromycin estolate is liver toxic. Hence the erythromycin is contra-indicated in patients with liver disease. Careful consideration is necessary for use of erythromycins in liver impaired patients.

The patient is advised to follow the following guidelines:

- Take the medicine with full glass of water 1 hour before or 2 hour after food (enteric coated preparations may be taken with meals).
- Do not take with fruit juice.
- Do not miss the dose. Take at evenly spaced times to keep a constant level of drug in body fluids. If it is time for next dose, skip the missed dose. Do not double the dose.
- Complete the full course of the medicine even if you feel better.
- Take the medicine on medical advice only.
- Do not use skin preparations of this medicine near eyes, nose, mouth, or other mucous membranes.

Complete the course of medicine.
Adhere to medication schedule.

Azithromycin: Azithromycin is more effective than erythromycin against certain infections. A single dose of azithromycin is used in the treatment of uncomplicated genital Chlamydia and trachoma. The adverse effects are similar to erythromycin but fewer gastrointestinal effects. Careful consideration is necessary for its use in liver impaired patients. The safe and effective user guidelines are:

- The usual adult dose is 500 mg once a day for most common infections.
- Take the medicine with full glass of water 1 hour before or 2 hour after food (Do not use antacids as they decrease the absorption of azithromycin).
- Do not miss the dose. Take at evenly spaced times to keep a constant level of drug in body fluids. If it is time for next dose, skip the missed dose. Do not double the dose.
- Complete the full course of the medicine even if you feel better.
- Promptly report the adverse effects either to your doctor or pharmacist.
- Take the medicine on medical advice only.

(d) Cephalosporins

Because of similar chemical structure, cephalosporins have spectrum of activities similar to ampicillin and similar mechanism of action as penicillins. They are powerful antibiotics against many different kinds of bacteria but often expensive. They can be used for pneumonia, urinary tract infection, typhoid, gut or pelvic infections, bone infections and meningitis. The common medicines of this category are cefazolin, cephalexin, cephradine, cefurazine, cefoxitin, ceftriaxone, cefotaxime and ceftazidime. Some are administered as injection to prevent infections before, during, and after surgery. However, cephalosporins are of no value in cold, flue or other viral infections.

Complete the course of medicine.
Adhere to medication schedule.

The common side effects are mild diarrhoea, nausea and vomiting, sore mouth or tongue, stomach cramp. One must report the side effects like abdominal or stomach cramps and severe pain; watery or severe diarrhoea; unusual bleeding or bruising to the treating doctor. The cephalosporins may also cause anaphylactic shock though rare. The safe and effective use guidelines:

- Take the medicines as prescribed by your doctor. Adhere to the dosing schedule.
- Do not miss the dose. Take at evenly spaced times to keep a constant level of drug in body fluids. If it is time for next dose, skip the missed dose. Do not double the dose.
- Complete the full course of the medicine even if you feel better.
- Promptly report the adverse effects either to your doctor or pharmacist.
- Tell your doctor, if you have any kidney problem. It may be necessary to reduce the dose.
- Take oral cephalosporins at least one hour before or 2 hours after meals for maximum benefits. However, if you experience gastric irritation, take them with meals.

- If you are taking other antibiotics like tetracyclines, erythromycins, chloramphenicol; take cephalosporins at least one hour before these medicines.
- Do not take alcohol in any form at least 72 hours (3 days) of treatment with some cephalosporins.
- Take curd or butter milk with your meal to prevent intestinal super infection resulting from suppression of normal bacterial flora.

(e) Quinolone Group Antibiotics

Ciprofloxacin and Norfloxacin are two common antibiotics of this group. Like other antibiotics, they are of no value in colds, flu or other viral infections. There are many other medicines in this group. But gatifloxacin is recently banned from use.

Ciprofloxacin is useful in the treatment of gastroenteritis including cholera; typhoid; gonorrhoea; meningitis; respiratory tract infections, urinary tract infections, bone and joint infections and many other infections. As ciprofloxacin is believed to cause arthropathy in weight bearing joints, it is not recommended in children and growing adolescents. It may impair the ability to perform skilled jobs like operating machineries or driving. Ciprofloxacin is available as tablets and injections. The safe and effective use guidelines are:

- The usual adult dose is 250-750 mg twice daily.
- Take the medicine preferably 2 hours after meals.
- Do not miss the dose. Take at evenly spaced times to keep a constant level of drug in body fluids. If it is time for next dose, skip the missed dose. Do not double the dose.
- Complete the full course of the medicine even if you feel better.
- Do not use in children unless the doctor specifically recommends.
- Avoid exposure to excessive sunlight (discontinue if photosensitivity occurs).
- Drink plenty of fluid to prevent crystalluria.
- Avoid antacids (also iron and calcium) during use of ciprofloxacin. If necessary, take them 2 hours before or 6 hours after ciprofloxacin.
- Avoid high alert and hazardous activities like driving or handling heavy machineries as the medicine may cause dizziness, light headedness or drowsiness.
- Avoid breast feeding.

Norfloxacin is available as tablets and primarily used in the treatment of urinary tract infection. It is also used in the treatment of uncomplicated gonorrhoea, gastroenteritis, and traveller's diarrhoea. The medicine should be used cautiously in patients with kidney disease or kidney malfunctioning. Patients with a history of seizures may have increased chances of seizures while taking this medicine. There are many medicines which interfere with functioning of Norfloxacin. Antacids and sucralfate (used in peptic ulcers) may decrease the effectiveness of Norfloxacin. On the other hand, Norfloxacin increases the chances of side effects from theophyline (anti-asthma drug). The common side effects of Norfloxacin are: abdominal or stomach pain or upset; constipation; diarrhoea; dizziness; drowsiness; headache; light headedness; loss of appetite; nausea or vomiting; and trouble in sleeping.

Complete the course of medicine. Adhere to medication schedule. Avoid excessive exposure to sunlight.

Drug	Indications (assuming causative bacteria are sensitive)
Ciprofloxacin	Abdominal infections, acute sinusitis, bone and joint infections, gonorrhea, infectious diarrhea, plague, pneumonia, chronic prostatitis, skin infections, typhoid fever, urinary tract infections
Norfloxacin	Urinary tract infection, urethral and cervical gonorrhea, prostatitis
Ofloxacin	Acute pelvic inflammatory disease, community-acquired pneumonia, gonorrhea, prostatitis, skin infections, sudden worsening of chronic bronchitis due to a bacterial infection, urinary tract infections
Levofloxacin	Acute sinusitis, hospital- and community-acquired pneumonia, plague, chronic prostatitis, skin infections, sudden worsening of chronic bronchitis due to a bacterial infection, urinary tract infections
Gemifloxacin	Community-acquired (as opposed to hospital-acquired) pneumonia, sudden worsening of chronic bronchitis due to a bacterial infection
Moxifloxacin	Abdominal infections, acute sinusitis, community-acquired pneumonia, plague, skin infections, sudden worsening of chronic bronchitis due to a bacterial infection

Gemifloxacin and Moxifloxacin have higher risks of adverse events compared to others of the group. Gemifloxacin is associated with higher rate of rash and QT prolongation. Moxifloxacinis not more effective than others but can cause QT prolongation.

This group of antibiotics are known to cause blood sugar disturbances (high blood sugar / low blood sugar) and a range of mental health conditions. Low blood sugar level, also known as hypoglycaemia, can lead to comma. The mental health side effects: disturbances in attention, disorientation, agitation, nervousness, memory impairment, serious disturbances in mental abilities (delirium).

This group of antibacterial drugs is usually not of first choice drugs as they have strong association with serious adverse events: tendon injury, diarrhea caused by *Clostridium difficile*, worsening muscle weakness especially in patients with myasthenia gravis, peripheral neuropathy, QT prolongation and fetal damage.

The fluoroquinolone group of antibacterials should be avoided in patients who already have some degree of QT prolongation, have hypokalemia or are taking other drugs that cause QT prolongation.

The safe and effective use guidelines are:

- Take with full glass of water in empty stomach (at least one hour before or two hours after meals).
- Do not miss any dose and take at evenly spaced time to maintain appropriate drug level. If it is time for next dose, skip the missed dose. Do not double the dose.
- Drink plenty of water during the medication period.
- Take full course of treatment even if you feel better after taking medicines for few days.
- Do not take antacids and sucralfate along with Norfloxacin. They should be taken at least 2 to 3 hours after Norfloxacin.
- Avoid excessive exposure to sunlight. Eyes and skins become more sensitive to sunlight. It is advisable to use sunglasses and protective clothing. The use of sun screening agents is also advised.
- Avoid high alert and hazardous activities like driving or handling heavy machineries as the medicine may cause dizziness, light headedness or drowsiness.

(f) Metronidazole

Metronidazole is useful in gut infections caused by amoebas, giardia and certain bacteria and sometimes for diarrhoea caused by taking antibiotics. It is useful in certain vaginal infections. The diarrhoea or dysentery caused by amoebas are characterized by frequent stools with much mucous and sometimes blood. There may be gut cramps. Amoebic dysentery is best treated with Metronidazole with diloxanide furoate. The amoebiasis is caused by the ingestion of cysts (*Entamoeba histolytica*) from contaminated food or drink. Giardasis is caused by oral ingestion of *Giardia* cysts. The stools are often yellow and frothy, but without blood or mucous. Trichomoniasis is a vaginal infection. Patients and their sexual partners too require treatment with Metronidazole.

Complete the course of medicine.
Adhere to medication schedule.

Metronidazole is available as tablets, suspensions and injections. The dose of Metronidazole is different for different conditions. The usual adult dose for amoebic dysentery is 250 mg to 500 mg three times a day for 5 to 10 days; for giardasis it is 2 gram once daily for three days; and for urogenital trichomoniasis it is 2 gram as single dose or 400-500 mg twice daily for seven days. The common side effects are diarrhoea; dizziness or light headedness; headache; loss of appetite; nausea or vomiting; stomach pain or cramps. However, the patient should report the experience of numbness, tingling, pain, or weakness in hands or feet to their doctors.

The patient should look into the following guidelines for safe and effective use of this medicine:

- Take medicine with meals to minimize gastric irritation.
- Do not drink alcohol in any form as this may cause severe nausea. Avoid alcohol for at least 48 hours after the last dose.
- Avoid during pregnancy especially during first three months of pregnancy.

- Tell your doctor, if you have medical problems like blood disease, epilepsy, heart disease, liver disease. Metronidazole may make blood disease worse; it may increase the chances of seizures; and patients with liver disease may have increased side effects.
- Do not miss the dose. Take at evenly spaced times to keep a constant level of drug in body fluids. If it is time for next dose, skip the missed dose. Do not double the dose.
- Complete the full course of the medicine even if you feel better.
- Practice good hygiene of washing hands after toileting and before handling, preparing or eating food.

(g) Phasing out of Antibiotics as Growth Promoters!

"We are moving to a post – antibiotic era where the pipeline of new antibiotic is virtually dry…the cupboard is nearly bare" warns World Health Organization. A British economist predicts "2 million Indians at risk of dying every year by 2050" due to antibiotic resistance. The antibiotic resistance, though a natural phenomenon, is global public health threat. The miracle medicines of today may not be useful tomorrow. Just because of this the pharmaceutical companies are not showing much interest in developing new antibiotics. Consequence of resistance is increased frequency of treatment failure including deaths and increased severity of infection.

While many factors including inappropriate use of antibiotics in human health are responsible for exacerbated development of resistance, theover use of antibiotics in farming sector is a major contributing factor. Agriculture or animal use of antibiotics is more extensive than human usage globally. It is estimated that the consumption of antibiotics in farms sector to grow from 63,200 tons in 2010 to 105,600 tons in 2030, an increase of two-third. The antibiotics are widely deployed on industrial scale farms not just to treat sick animals but to prevent diseases and promote faster growth. The history of use of antibiotics in promoting animal growth goes back to the discovery of 1950. The scientists in New York discovered that adding antibiotics to livestock feed accelerated animals' growth and cost less than conventional feed supplements. Since then worldwide sub-therapeutic dose of antibiotics are continued to be in practice to enhance animal growth or to improve feed efficiency in spite of warning of bacterial resistance. With increased population and growing demand of animal proteins, antibiotics are increasingly used to raise food producing animals in intensive production.

The use of antibiotics in animal food production poses a big threat to human health in many ways. The resistant strains of bacteria spread from animals and / or the environment (ground water, surface water, soil) to humans. Direct animal to human transmission of resistance, animal food to human transmission of resistance, food-borne outbreak of infection, and parallel trends in antibiotic use in animals and related antibiotic resistance in humans are the ways human health is affected by antibiotic use in livestock. Farmers working with cattle, pigs, and poultry are at much higher risk of infection with the resistant bacteria. The human consumption of food carrying antibiotic resistant bacteria can lead to drug resistant infection. The antibiotic resistance is not only affecting human health but puts animal health at risk too. "The antibiotic over use and resistance would have enormous adverse impact on rural lively hoods and food security" warns United Nations Food and Agriculture Organization.

There is an interesting history too. In 1961, on the set of 'Cleopatra' actress Elizabeth Taylor developed a highly lethal lung infection caused by staph bacteria. But staph was resistant to miracle drug of the time, penicillin. A new synthetic form of penicillin, methicillin, was just developed to save her life. Now most of the staph bacteria are resistant to methicillin and methicillin resistant *Staphylococcus aureus* (MRSA) are widespread. Now it is believed that human strain of MRSA originated in livestock. The use of avoparcin, an antibiotic, as growth promoter in food animals in Europe resulted in development of vancomycin resistant enterococci and subsequent colonization in human intestine. Vancomycin resistance is a cause of concern as it is often the last line antibiotic for treatment of some hospital acquired infections.

One study conducted by Delhi based civil society reported that 40% of poultry samples contained one or more of the five antibiotics tested: enrofloxacin, doxycycline, ciprofloxacin, oxytetracycline and chlortetracycline. The situation in other countries is not much different. Realizing the threat of overuse of antibiotics not for therapeutic purpose but for promoting growth of food animals, the Consumer International called for stop using meats from animals routinely administered antibiotics used in human medicines. On this World Consumer Rights Day (March 15), consumer international urged the people to pressurize the food industry to stop using antibiotics in their meat supply chain. Antibiotics Off The Menu!

World Health Organization recommends that critically important antimicrobials identified should be prudently used both in human and veterinary medicines. The antibiotics like carbapenems, lipopeptides, oxazolidinones and any new antibiotic discovered should not be used in animals, plants and aqua culture. Reducing the use of antibiotics in agriculture is an urgent and necessary step towards tackling this public health crisis.The Netherlands has taken lead by reducing almost 60% of drug use in livestock sector. While continuing the prudent use of antibiotics for treating infections in animals, the general use of antibiotics particularly for growth promotion of live stocks must be avoided. The sensitization of farmers and the veterinary professionals, improvement in hygiene, disease prevention and regulatory strategies, along with good nutrition to improve overall health of live stocks are critical in reducing the overuse of antibiotics. A priority attention is necessary in the interest of public health. Misuse of antibiotics in animals endanger human health!

(h) Avoid Antibiotics that Lower the Blood Glucose to a Dangers Level in Diabetics!

Diabetes continues to be a concern in our society and the health system as well. The annual number of deaths in India due to diabetes has increased more than two folds between 1990 and 2010. With increasing incidences, the world has given India the title "Diabetes capital of World". Oral hypoglycaemic medicines are the choice for managing Type 2 diabetes if glycemic target are not achieved with modification of diet, maintenance of a healthy body weight and regular physical activity.

Hypoglycaemia is a commonly recognised adverse effect associated with insulin and sulphonyl urea medicines [glipizide or glyburide]. This develops suddenly with symptoms of nervousness, trembling, weakness, sweating, intense hunger, palpitation and disorientation; and in extreme case loss of consciousness. Elderly patients, patients who have diabetes for long time, have kidney damage, use more than one diabetes medicine, involved in extensive glycemic control activities, or have problems with memory are more likely to develop hypoglycaemia. Severe hypoglycaemia is also associated with increased risks of cardiovascular events like heart attacks and stroke, cognitive impairment, dementia and death.

The recent research published in Journal of American Medical Association (JAMA) Internal Medicine showed that five antibiotics: ciprofloxacin, clarithromycin, levofloxacin, Metronidazole, and cotrimoxazole are associated with increased risk of severe hypoglycaemia in patients treated with sulphonylurea. The increased greatest risk is found to be with clarithromcin and least risk with the use of ciprofloxacin. The researchers concluded that the drug (Antibiotics)-drug (glipizide or glyburide) interaction is the cause of hypoglycaemia. Clarithromycin increases the drug level of sulphonyl urea; Levofloxacin increases the drug action and increases the drug level; Metronidazole interferes with drug metabolism; Cotrimoxazole interferes with drug metabolism; and ciprofloxacin enhances drug action. The problem of drug – drug interaction is more likely in our country when the diabetic patients self medicate with antibiotics. Many times the use of these antibiotics is not necessary. The patients need to be discouraged self medication especially with antibiotics in their own interest and in the interest of the community.

The physicians and the pharmacists must realize that the avoidance of serious life threatening hypoglycaemia is the key component of successful diabetes management. If the diabetic patients, already with glipizide or glyburide, need antibiotic therapy, avoid using the antibiotics (antibiotics includes other antibacterial medicines too) described earlier. Alternative antibiotics are available. The patients should also be educated on the symptoms, danger and immediate management of hypoglycaemia.

CHAPTER 54

Anti-Malaria Medicines

(a) Fighting Malaria with Artesunate Combination Therapy

Malaria accounts for over one million deaths and up to one million cases a year worldwide. This is a protozoal disease caused by, alone or in combination, *Plasmodium vivax, Plasmodium falciparum, Plasmodium oval and Plasmodium malariae.* The parasites are inoculated into human beings by a female anopheline mosquito bites. The first symptoms of malaria are non-specific and they include fever, chills, sweating, muscle and joint pain, abdominal pain, diarrhoea, nausea, vomiting, loss of appetite. These are the common symptoms of uncomplicated malaria.

The parasite has the potential to develop resistance against the medicines used to treat it. Once very effective and widely used affordable medicine, chloroquine, becomes ineffective because of increasing resistance. The resistance to other anti-malarial medicines is also rapidly developing. The biggest challenge for treating malaria is to prevent development of resistance to the effective medicines. The development and discovery of Artemisinin and its derivatives provides a solution. Artemisinin based combination therapy (ACT) is now recognized as best current treatment for uncomplicated falciparum malaria. The World Health Organization (WHO) has recommended this combination therapy in its recent guidelines for treatment of malaria.

The treatment goal should direct towards the dual objectives: cure of infection and to prevent the emergence and spread of resistance to anti-malarials. Tolerability and adverse effect profile are also important consideration in selection of anti-malarials. However, saving life should be the main criteria in treatment of severe malaria. Widespread and indiscriminate use of anti-malarials places a strong selective pressure on malaria parasite to develop high level of resistance. Resistance can be prevented or at least its onset slowed down considerably by combining anti-malarials with different mechanisms of actions. But they should have high cure rates through full adherence to correct regimens.

Complete the course of medicine.
Adhere to medication schedule.

The combination therapy is more effective as the different medicines work through different mechanisms. If the resistance develops for one drug, then the other will kill parasites. The combinations are independently effective. On the other hand, the combination therapy too also has some disadvantages like increased risk of adverse effects and high cost.

Artemisinin and its derivatives (artesunate, artemether, artemotil, dihydroartemisinin) kill the malaria parasites quickly and the patient recovers fast. The WHO recommends that artemisinin be part of combination therapy (ACT) together with another anti-malarial. ACTs are unlikely to have problems of resistance at least in near future. The ACTs are well tolerated and active against all species of *Plasmodium.* The following combinations are recommended by WHO: artemether – lumefantrine, artesunate – amodiaquine, artesunate – mefloquine, artesunate – sulphadoxine and pyrimethamine (SP). At present some are only available as combination medicine and others would be made available as combinations in due course of time. The country guideline or the individual physician decides which combinations would be best suitable for the individual patients. The body weight, age of the patient and severity of infection, resistance pattern prevailing are the determining factor for the type of therapy, dose and duration. Remember: "Combination therapy makes it harder for the malaria parasite to become resistant".

It is dangerous not to use malaria medicines correctly. It could be expensive to use the medicines incorrectly. The patients may become serious requiring costly medicines or hospitalisation. The incorrect use may contribute to resistance development and the effective medicines of today may not be useful tomorrow. Here are few practical tips for appropriate use of anti-malarial medicines:

- Make sure that you know the relevant information about the medicines prescribed or advised: How to take or use and the likely adverse effects etc. Discuss these with your doctor or pharmacist.

- Inform your doctor if you are pregnant. Mefloquine needs to be avoided.
- Never use Artemisinin or its derivatives alone. Use with another effective malarial medicine.
- If all or part of a dose is vomited within one hour of swallowing, the same amount should be given immediately.
- Take oral choroquine after meals to help prevent nausea and vomiting.
- Adhere to the dosage schedule as prescribed or advised.
- Keep the medicines beyond the reach of children.

(b) Other Anti-Malarial Medicines

The effective treatment of malaria aims at providing complete cure of malaria cases and preventing development of drug resistance through rational treatment. The uncomplicated malaria cases caused by *Plasmodium vivax* can be treated with chloroquine and primaquine. However, ACT (Artemisinin Combination Therapy) is recommended for uncomplicated *plasmodium falciparum* cases. The complicated malaria requires parenteral therapy.

Chloroquine: Chloroquine is a rapidly acting drug and is safe and effective too. A three day course by mouth with fourteen day course of primaquine is recommended for vivax malaria cases. [Chloroquine is also useful in the treatment of rheumatoid arthritis and amoebiasis]. Chloroquine is available as oral syrup, tablet and injection. Guidelines for safe and effective use:

- Take after meals to minimize nausea and vomiting. If part or all a dose is vomited, take the same amount immediately.
- Do not expose to excessive sunlight.
- If you experience blurred vision, increased sensitivity to light, hearing loss, pronounced gastric disturbance, or muscle weakness, immediately report to your doctor.
- Complete the course and do not stop without your doctor's advice.

Complete the course of medicine.
Adhere to medication schedule.

Primaquine: Primaquine is often used with fast acting anti-malarial, chloroquine. It is contraindicated (not to be used) in G6PD deficient patients, infants and pregnant women. Primaquine can lead to haemolytic anaemia in G6PD deficient patients. It is advisable to screen the patients for possible G6PD deficiency. The useful guidelines:

- Complete the entire course of therapy.
- Take medicine with meals to minimize gastric irritation.

- Do not take with gastric antacids.
- Check urine colour and report if urine darkens, becomes tinged with red, or decreases in volume.

Dosage schedule for uncomplicated Malaria (*Plasmodium vivax)*

Age in years	**Tablet Chloroquine (150 mg base)**			**Tablet Primaquine (2.5 mg base)**
	Day 1	Day 2	Day 3	Day 1 to Day 14
15 and above	4 (single dose)	4 (single dose)	2 (single dose)	6 (single dose)

CHAPTER 55

Anti-Tuberculosis Medicines

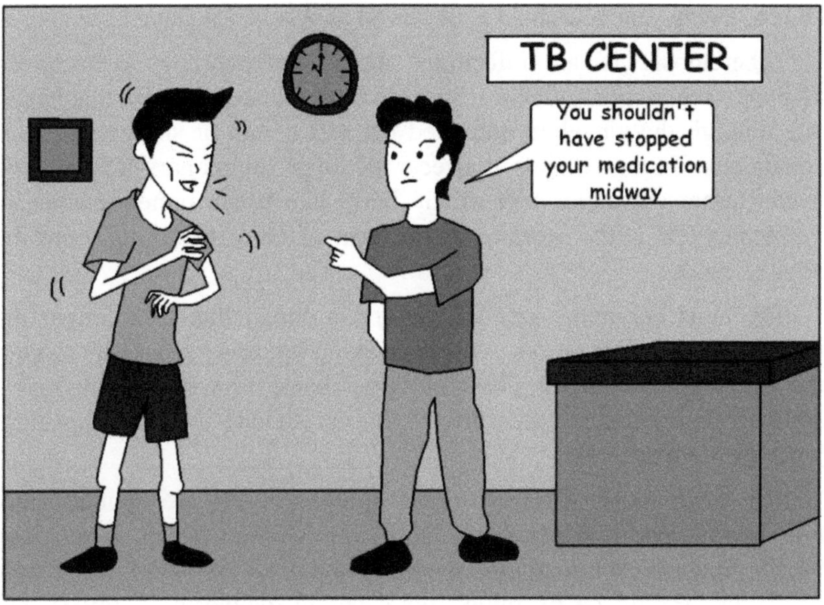

(a) DOTS: a Sure Cure for Tuberculosis

In India today, two deaths occur every three minutes from tuberculosis (TB). A single patient can infect 10 or more persons in a year. India is the highest burden country globally accounting for one-fifth of global incidence. These sound alarming. But there is a sure cure for TB, the DOTS. Every year March 24 is observed as World TB Day.

Tuberculosis is an infectious disease caused by a bacterium, *Mycobacterium tuberculosis.* It spreads from a disease person to a healthy one through the air when untreated patients cough or sneeze. It is very contagious. Though mainly it affects the lungs (pulmonary tuberculosis), it can affect any other part of the body like brain, bones, glands etc. Pulmonary TB is the most common form of TB constituting more than 85% of cases.

The most common signs of TB are: a cough that lasts longer than two weeks and often worse just after waking up; fever especially rising in the evening; pain in the chest or upper back; loss of weight; loss of appetite. In advanced cases the symptoms include coughing up blood, voice grows hoarse etc.

The main tools of diagnosis of pulmonary TB are sputum smear microscopy, chest X ray, and culture of *Mycobacterium tuberculosis* bacilli. Sputum examination is the key diagnostic tool and three samples of sputum should be examined for accurate diagnosis. X ray is more expensive and less accurate, though essential for some patients.

Complete the course of medicines even if you feel better. Adhere to medication schedule. This is in the best interest of you, your family and the community.

DOTS is directly observed treatment, short course. It is the most effective way to ensure cure. The treatment aims to cure, prevent development of resistance, decrease infection and break the chain of transmission of infection whilst minimising the side effects of medicines. Under revised National Tuberculosis Programme, DOT medicines are supplied free.

Drug	Dose	Number of Tablets each dose
Isoniazid	600 mg	2 tabs
Rifampicin	450 mg	1 tab (if patient weight is more than 60 kg, additional 150 mg)
Pyrazinamide	1500 mg	2 tabs
Ethambutol	1200 mg	2 tabs
Streptomycin	750 mg (if patient is more than 50 years and those who weigh less than 30 kg, dose is 500 mg)	---------

Based on diagnosis, the patients are grouped into three categories for treatment. The medicines are supplied in patient wise boxes containing full course of treatment and packed in blister packs. The patient wise boxes have a colour code indicating the category: Red for category I, Blue for category II and Green for category III. In each category treatment there are two phases: intensive phase and continuation phase. In directly observed treatment, a health worker or another person who is not a family member watches as the patient swallows the medicines in their presence. The minimum treatment period is 6 months and may go up to 8 months depending upon the category. During intensive phase of treatment the medicines are to be taken by the patients under direct supervision. In the continuation phase at least the first dose is to be taken by the patient under direct supervision and next two doses of the week are given to the patients for self administration. Patients are encouraged to bring the blister pack of the previous week of treatment as a measure to check whether the doses are taken or not. A treatment card is prepared and a copy is given to each patient along with patient's medicine box.

Though anti-tuberculosis medicines are generally safe, side effects may occur in some cases. Isoniazid can damage the liver. Person who develops the signs of hepatitis needs to stop taking medicine and report to the physician. Rifampicin too can cause liver damage. It can cause urine, tears, faeces, saliva, and sweat orange coloured. But there is no reason to concern. Pyrazinamide may cause swollen and painful joints. Ethambutol may cause eye pain or damage. It should be stopped if eye problem or blurred vision appears. The vision gets better slowly after the medication is stopped. Streptomycin may cause deafness. If the ringing of ears or deafness begins, the medicine is to be stopped and doctor be consulted. The side effects are one of the main reasons for not continuing the full course of treatment when patients start feeling better after one or two months of treatment.

The general guidelines for using anti-TB medicines:

- Adhere to the treatment protocol as given under DOTS.
- Be proactive in using medicines, though the health worker will try to ensure your adherence to medication schedule.
- Continue the treatment even if you feel better after a few months of treatment.
- If you experience the side effects described above, report to your DOTS provider or doctor immediately. Your doctor will suggest alternate regimen.
- Tell your doctor if you have kidney problem, the doctor will adjust the dose in such patients.
- Never take these medicines without doctor's advice.

Few patient centric approaches are initiated:

- **Interested private pharmacies can stock Government Supply anti-TB medicines and become the DOTS provider. The patients can get their medicine from these pharmacies.**
- **New daily regiment is introduced.**
- **Nutritional support of Rs. 500/- per month to each patient through direct benefit transfer.**

(b) DOTS – Plus for Multi Drug Resistant TB

While World Health Organization's recommended Directly Observed Treatment – Short Course (DOTS) is a sure cure for Tuberculosis (TB), the non adherence to the treatment protocol leads to treatment failure and emergence of multi drug resistant tuberculosis (MDR-TB). One of the readers of my column wanted to know on the use of medicines in the treatment of MDR-TB.

MDR-TB is defined as an infection caused by *Mycobacterium tuberculosis* resistant to the most active anti-TB drugs: Isoniazid and Rifampicin. The TB organism may or may not have resistance to other anti-TB drugs. MDR – TB can be diagnosed in a specialized laboratory. The treatment of such condition not only requires longer duration of treatment but the medicines used for the treatment are more expensive and toxic. There is still further serious type of TB called extensively drug resistant TB (XDR-TB). XDR-TB is defined as TB where the infective TB organism is not only resistant to isoniazid and rifampicin but also resistant to any of the fluoroquinolones (ciprofloxacin, norfloxacin, gatifloxacin etc.) and any one of the second line injectable drugs (amikacin, kanamycin, or capreomycin). MDR – TB can be transformed into XDR – TB through inadequate or interrupted treatment with second line anti-TB drugs.

Though drug resistant TB is a global issue with half a million new cases of MDR-TB and 40,000 new cases of XDR –TB are emerging each year, India is second only to China in terms of prevalence of MDR-TB. It is not fully explored the extent of problems of MDR-TB and XDR – TB in our country. The government of India advocates the use of DOTS-Plus service for the effective treatment of MDR-TB. DOTS-Plus programme has shown good treatment outcomes compared to treatment followed outside of structured treatment programmes.

Complete the course of medicines even if you feel better. Adhere to medication schedule. This is in the best interest of you, your family and the community.

The accurate diagnosis and effective treatment of patients with MDR-TB is crucial to improve treatment outcome, reduce deaths and prevent generation of XDR-TB. Drug resistance is suspected and diagnosed from the history of prior treatment and through culture and drug susceptibility testing from quality assured laboratories. The Revised National TB Control Programme (RNTCP) of Government of India is in the process of establishing the accredited laboratories. Detection of XDR TB is technically very difficult and only done at a very small number of laboratories.

The DOTS-Plus programme has standardized regimen for the treatment of MDR-TB. The duration of treatment is divided into two phases: at least 6 months of intensive phase, which may be extended to 9 months for patients who have a positive culture result taken at 4th month of treatment and a minimum of 18 months of continuation phase following the intensive phase.

Phase	Medicines	Period of treatment
Intensive phase	Kanamycin, Ofloxacin, Ethionamide, Cycloserine, Pyrazinamide and Ethambutol	6 to 9 months
Extensive phase	Ofloxacin, Ethambutol, Cycloserine and Ethionamide.	18 months

Kanamycin is an injectable antibiotic which should be used in the same time each day. Diarrhoea, nausea, pain, redness or swelling at injection site are common side effects. If severe side effects such as allergic reactions, decreased urination, hearing loss, ringing or roaring in the ears, vaginal irritations or discharge occur, it is to be reported to the treating doctor immediately. Ofloxacin is a fluoroquinolone group anti-bacterial drug used in conjunction with other anti-TB medicines. One needs to avoid its use during pregnancy. It may cause dizziness and light headedness. One has to be careful when driving or operating hazardous machinery. Other medicines like antacids, vitamins may influence the activity of ofloxacin. Separation of their administration by 2 to 4 hours is advisable. Ethionamide should be taken with or after meals to prevent stomach upset. Diabetes type-2 may be difficult to control while taking ethionamide. Patients with severe liver disease may have increased side effects. Often Vit B_6 (pyridoxine) is advised to reduce its side effects. Action of cycloserine may get affected in presence of other medical problems such as alcohol abuse, convulsive disorder, kidney disease, and mental disorders. It increases the risk of seizure and dose adjustment is necessary in kidney disease. Cycloserine may cause anxiety, mental depression, or psychosis. Pyrazinamide may worsen or cause a gout attack, and patients with severe side effects experience increased side effects. Ethambutol may cause blurred vision, red-green color blindness, or changes in urine elimination. However, these visual alterations will disappear within several weeks or months after the medicine is discontinued.

General guidelines:

- Do not try to self medicate with these drugs. They are second line of anti-TB medicines and are to be used under medical advice only after diagnosis as MDR TB.
- To clear up your TB completely, you must keep taking these medicines for the full time of treatment, even if you begin to feel better.
- Do not miss doses. Consult your doctor what is to be done as it may require rescheduling your dosage regimen.
- While taking ofloxacin: drink plenty of fluids; separate doses of antacids, vitamins and ofloxacin by 2 hours; avoid prolonged exposure to direct sunlight and use sunscreen agents when outdoor; careful while operating hazardous machineries or driving as one may feel dizziness and light headedness.
- Take ethionamide, cycloserine after meals to reduce stomach upset.
- Do not drink alcohol, as it may increase the risk of seizure in presence of cycloserine. If you feel depressed or thought of suicide, consult your doctor immediately. This could be the side effect of cycloserine.
- These medicines are very toxic. Keep out of reach of children.
- All these medicines have several side effects. Report back immediately if you do experience an unusual event.
- Keep follow up appointments with your doctor or health centre.

(c) DOTS for Paediatric Tuberculosis

Tuberculosis (TB) is one of the major diseases afflicting children throughout the world, with approximately 1 million new cases and 400,000 deaths every year. Though good data on prevalence of all types of TB in children is difficult to obtain, it can be anywhere around 10 percent of total TB cases. Paediatric TB is more common in females while the adult TB in males. Extra Pulmonary TB is more common in children than adults. Earlier TB in children was a neglected issue as most paediatric cases have limited infectiousness.

The pulmonary TB in children is suspected when they are presented with: fever and/or cough for more than 3 weeks; with or without weight loss or no weight gain; and history of contact with a suspected or diagnosed case of active TB in last 2 years. The diagnosis of TB in children is based on clinical condition, sputum examination where ever possible, chest X ray, Mantoux test and history of contact. Children who are most at risk are those who: have had household contact with a newly diagnosed smear positive case, are aged less than five years, are living with HIV, and are severly malnourished. Children showing neurological symptoms like irritability, refusal to feed, headache, vomiting or altered sensorium may be suspected to have meningitis TB.

The main problem associated with the paediatric TB is difficulty in diagnosis and treatment. The treatment regimens are different from that of adults, non availability of all anti Tb medicines in paediatric formulations and safety of all medicines in children. The Revised National Tuberculosis Control Programme has designed the dosage regimen based on body weight for all children less than 6 years of age. For all children above 6 years, the same regimen is recommended as for adults.

Give the complete course of medicines even if child feels better. Adhere to medication schedule.

- The two key indicators which alert the suspicion of TB are: history of close contact with TB; and chronic cough, fever and weight loss.
- Take your children to RNTCP centre for diagnosis and treatment.
- Children usually tolerate the TB medicines well and serious side effects are uncommon.
- Ensure strict adherence of dosage schedule for your children. Condition of your children may improve after few weeks of treatment, but continue treatment for full course for complete cure.

(d) New anti-TB Drugs for Resistant TB

Bedaquiline 100 mg Tablet [for MDR-TB]

Bedaquiline is recently approved by the Government of India for use as part of combination therapy of pulmonary tuberculosis due to multi-drug resistant *Mycobacterium tuberculosis*. This should be used when an effective treatment cannot be provided. US FDA has approved this drug in December 2012 under fast track basis. This is the first US FDA approved tuberculosis drug in last 40 years.

Having limited data on safety and efficacy of the drug, the World Health Organization (WHO) has the following interim recommendations:

- To be added to only WHO recommended regimen in adult MDR – TB patients;
- Treatment should be offered under closely monitored conditions;
- Treatment is meant only for adults (18 years and above). Special precaution for persons of 65 years or older and adults with HIV. Use in pregnant women and children is not advisable;
- Should be used with caution in patients with co-morbidities (diabetes), or persons with alcohol or substance abuse;
- There is need of clinical monitoring and management of co-morbidities (especially cardiac and liver diseases);
- To be used for a maximum duration of 6 months and at suggested dosing (400 mg daily for the first 2 weeks, followed by 200 mg three times per week for the remaining 22 weeks);
- There should be system to ensure early detection and timely reporting of adverse events using active pharmacovigilance methods (cohort event monitoring);
- Must not be added alone to a failing regiment;
- Resistance to the drug should be monitored; and
- Duly informed decision making process by the patients should be followed.

Adverse events (AE): The most frequently reported are nausea, arthralgia, headache, hyperuricaemia, and vomiting. Additional AEs are in order of frequency: dizziness, increased transaminases, myalgia, diarrhoea and QT prolongation on electrocardiogram (ECG) and hepatic disorder. Limited clinical trial data showed higher incidences of deaths compared to placebo groups.

Efficacy: The proportion of subjects defined as cured at 120 weeks was 57.6 % in the bedaquiline arm versus 31.8% in the placebo arm.

[Source: The use of bedaquiline in the treatment of multi-drug resistant tuberculosis, Interim Policy Guidance, WHO, 2013)

Delamanid

The Government of India has recently approved this drug for the treatment of multi-drug resistant tuberculosis. The World Health Organization currently recommends that the drug may be added to the WHO recommended regimen in adults with Pulmonary MDR-TB with five conditions: proper patient inclusion, adherence to the principle of designing a WHO recommended MDR-TB regimen, close treatment monitoring, active pharmacovigilance and proper management of adverse drug reactions, and informed patient consent. Later, its use is also recommended for children and adolescents (6 years – 17 years) with multi drug or rifampicin resistant TB (MDR/RR-TB) who are not eligible for the shorter MDR-TB with similar conditions as specified for adults.

Dose:

For patients aged 6-11 years: 50 mg twice a day for 6 months;

For patients aged 12-17 years: 100 mg twice a day for 6 months;

For adult patients: 100 mg twice a day.

The medicine is to be taken after food.

Adverse Effects:

The common side effects are: nausea, vomiting and dizziness. Other important side effects include anxiety, pins and needles, and shaking. It may cause serious side effect: QT prolongation.

In view of these side effects, the patients need to be closely monitored.

CHAPTER 56

Anti-Asthma Medicines

(a) Beat the Wheeze

The asthma medicines are available for use either as oral dosage forms, as injections or as inhalation. The inhalation is preferred because of quick relief obtained from use of inhalers. There are two types of inhalers: aerosol inhalers commonly called as puffer and dry powder inhalers, called as rotahalers.

Aerosol inhalers require good coordination between the pressing down of the inhaler to release the dose and breathe in (both should be done at the same time). Study has reported that more than 80% of the patients do not use the inhalers correctly. The correct use of inhalers deposits only about 9% of inhaled particles (medicaments) from an aerosol into lungs. Incorrect inhaler technique can reduce drug delivery and efficacy. Because of prevalence of suboptimal inhalation technique many patients may need additional device that can improve delivery of medicaments to the airways. One of these special devices is spacer. More medication gets into the lungs when an aerosol inhaler is used with a spacer device.

A spacer is a special device shaped like a clear plastic football or tube. The aerosol medication is fired into the device and then medication is inhaled through a face mask or mouth piece. By placing the spacer between the aerosol inhaler's mouth piece and patient's mouth, the patient is permitted to separate the activation of the aerosol from inhalation by up to 3-5 seconds as the valve in the spacer opens when the patient inhales. The guidelines for use of spacers:

1. Assemble the spacer.
2. Remove the cap from the inhaler.
3. Shake the inhaler well.

4. Attach the inhaler to the end of spacer.
5. Place the mouth piece of the spacer in your mouth and close your lips around it.
6. Press down the inhaler to release a dose into the spacer.
7. Breathe in for about 4 seconds and hold it for around 10 seconds. Then breathe out.
8. To take additional dose, shake the inhaler and repeat the steps from 4 to 7.

The spacer helps maintaining better control of asthma compared to using just inhalers. The spacer too needs to be cleaned every one to two weeks. It should be washed in clean hot soapy water and allowed to drip dry.

Learn the use of these devices to get maximum benefits.

Dry powder inhalers are available in different forms but rotahalers are most common. Deep inhalation is required to get the medication into the lungs. The dry powder medications are enclosed in the hard gelatine capsule shells (known as rotacaps). The basic operation is to remove the dry powder medicaments from the capsule shells into the rotahalers and then inhale. The guidelines are:

- Remove the rotahaler from its container.
- Hold the rotahaler by mouth piece and twist the barrel in either direction until it stops.
- Put the rotacap into square hole with clear end first. Make sure that the top of the rotacap is level with top of the hole.
- Hold the rotahaler horizontally, twist barrel sharply forwards and backwards. This splits capsule into two. The capsule contents are now ready for inhalation.
- Breathe out slowly and completely.
- Keep rotahaler level and place the mouth piece over your tongue an dwell into your mouth. Close your lips around the mouth piece and tilt your head slightly backwards.
- Breathe in the powder quickly and deeply as you can.
- Hold breathe as long as you are comfortable and then remove the rotahaler from the mouth.

- If any powder is left, repeat steps 5 to 8.
- Open the rotahalers pulling two halves apart and discard the empty rotacap shell.
- Reassemble the rotahaler.
- If second dose is necessary, complete the whole process again.

It is necessary to keep the rotahaler always in its container to keep it clean. Keep it clean at least every two weeks in warm water. Dry it completely before putting them together.

The patient needs to learn the use of spacer or the rotahaler to get the maximum benefit out of such medications. They should ask their doctors or pharmacists. The children may find difficult to use inhalers or rotahalers. Spacers are of great help in such situation.

(b) Keep Inhalers Handy

Winter is perhaps the worst time for asthmatics. With winter setting in, the asthma patients need to gear themselves with keeping the asthma medications handy. Asthma is a disease of the respiratory system where people have sensitive airways in their lungs. When it happens, the airways become narrow making it hard for them to breathe.

Asthma is increasing in prevalence in our society. It is reported that around 15% of our population suffer from either a mild or severe form of asthma. The burden is believed to be more than 15 million in our country. The common symptoms of asthma are unproductive cough, wheezing (a fine whistling sound), chest tightness and sensation of shortness of breath.

There are three main factors that cause the airways to become narrow: the inside lining of the airways becomes red and swollen (inflammation), extra mucous may be produced, and the muscle around the airways tightens (bronchoconstriction). Asthma attacks are commonly caused by exposure to specific allergens, air pollutants, industrial chemicals, or infection. They can be caused by exercise too especially in cold air. Even the emotional factors can worsen the condition. The allergens usually responsible for asthma attacks are dust mites, pollen, animal fur and feathers. Sudden change of temperature and cold air of winter are known triggers of asthma. This time of the year being the deewali season, people get their homes renovated. Fumes from paints and dusts from carpentry too are problematic. Pollution and smoke produced during cracker bursting and firework display are often dreaded for asthmatic patients. In all such situations, the asthmatics do need to keep their inhalers handy.

Inhalers deliver medicines directly to the respiratory tract. Learn the use of inhalers to get maximum benefits.

The goal of medicine therapy is to control asthma symptoms, to reduce frequency of attacks, and severity of exacerbations, and to reverse air flow obstruction. Basically there are two groups of medicines used in the management of asthma (there are other categories of medicines too): use of bronchodilators and anti-inflammatory agents. The bronchodilators cause dilation of the airways and the anti-inflammatory agents reduce the inflammation in the airways. When there is little response to bronchodilators, the anti-inflammatory agents like steroids (corticosteroids) are advised to be used to quickly regain control of asthma. The asthma medicines can be: taken orally, by injection or by inhalation. Inhalation is preferred because quick relief can be obtained by this route.

With inhalation medication goes directly to the lungs and smaller doses may be necessary with fewer side effects. There are two types of inhalers: aerosol inhaler (puffer) and dry powder inhaler. The aerosol inhalers are more common. Asthma care depends on the proper use of medication and inhalers. Under treatment and suboptimal therapy are the major factors that contribute to morbidity and mortality.

Aerosol inhalers are pressurized package when pressed it releases one dose. They are also known as metered dose inhalers. Though earlier chlorofluorocarbons were used to build pressure in the inhaler, based on Montreal protocol the present day asthma inhalers are now environment friendly. To get maximum benefit from the use of inhalers, it is necessary that they are properly used. The following guidelines are helpful (most of the inhalers come with user guidelines and the patients need to read and follow):

1. Remove the plastic cap that covers the mouthpiece.
2. Shake the inhaler vigorously before taking each dose.
3. Breathe out as fully as you comfortably can.
4. Tilt the chin up and hold the inhalers upright keeping mouth piece in your mouth. Create a seal with your lips.
5. Breathe in deeply as you press down on the can with your index finger.
6. When you complete breathe in, hold your breath as long as you comfortably can.
7. Remove the inhaler from the mouth and replace the cover.

If you need more than one dose (puff), repeat the process from 2-6 after 1 minute of administering the first dose. If steroid inhaler is used, rinsing mouth after each use is necessary. The whole process requires good coordination between pressing down the canister and breathe in. When the coordination is a problem, inhalers can be used with a spacer device for ensuring more medication reaching lungs.

Like appropriate use of inhalers, it is important to maintain them. The inhalers should be cleaned daily. To do this, remove the can from the plastic case. Rinse the plastic case and cap in warm water preferably under running water. Dry thoroughly and replace the metal can into the case. Put the cap on the mouthpiece. This would keep the mouth piece free of particles and prevent clogging.

Here are few general guidelines for appropriate use of inhalers and proper management of your asthma:

- Do not self medicate. The types of medicines used to treat asthma attacks are quite strong. If used incorrectly, they may have an immediate and dangerous effect on the health of the user.
- Learn to use your inhalers correctly. Discuss with your doctor or pharmacist.
- Do not use more or less than the recommended dose without consulting your doctor.
- Regularly check that your inhaler is not empty.
- The inhalers are pressurized packs. Do not puncture. Do not discard them into fire too.
- Try to avoid the triggering factors that cause asthma or that worsen your asthma.
- If you experience any side effect of the medicine using, report to your doctor or pharmacist.

(c) Use of Spacers and Rotahalers in Asthma

The asthma medicines are available for use either as oral dosage forms, as injections or as inhalation. The inhalation is preferred because of quick relief obtained from use of inhalers. There are two types of inhalers: aerosol inhalers commonly called as puffer and dry powder inhalers, called as rotahalers.

Aerosol inhalers require good coordination between the pressing down of the inhaler to release the dose and breathe in (both should be done at the same time). Study has reported that more than 80% of the patients do not use the inhalers correctly. The correct use of inhalers deposits only about 9% of inhaled particles (medicaments) from an aerosol into lungs. Incorrect inhaler technique can reduce drug delivery and efficacy. Because of prevalence of suboptimal inhalation technique many patients may need additional device that can improve delivery of medicaments to the airways. One of these special devices is spacer. More medication gets into the lungs when an aerosol inhaler is used with a spacer device.

A spacer is a special device shaped like a clear plastic football or tube. The aerosol medication is fired into the device and then medication is inhaled through a face mask or mouth piece. By placing the spacer between the aerosol inhaler's mouth piece and patient's mouth, the patient is permitted to separate the activation of the aerosol from inhalation by up to 3-5 seconds as the valve in the spacer opens when the patient inhales. The guidelines for use of spacers:

1. Assemble the spacer.
2. Remove the cap from the inhaler.
3. Shake the inhaler well.
4. Attach the inhaler to the end of spacer.
5. Place the mouth piece of the spacer in your mouth and close your lips around it.
6. Press down the inhaler to release a dose into the spacer.
7. Breathe in for about 4 seconds and hold it for around 10 seconds. Then breathe out.
8. To take additional dose, shake the inhaler and repeat the steps from 4 to 7.

The spacer helps maintaining better control of asthma compared to using just inhalers. The spacer too needs to be cleaned every one to two weeks. It should be washed in clean hot soapy water and allowed to drip dry.

Learn the use of these devices to get maximum benefits.

Dry powder inhalers are available in different forms but rotahalers are most common. Deep inhalation is required to get the medication into the lungs. The dry powder medications are enclosed in the hard gelatine capsule shells (known as rotacaps). The basic operation is to remove the dry powder medicaments from the capsule shells into the rotahalers and then inhale. The guidelines are:

1. Remove the rotahaler from its container.
2. Hold the rotahaler by mouth piece and twist the barrel in either direction until it stops.
3. Put the rotacap into square hole with clear end first. Make sure that the top of the rotacap is level with top of the hole.
4. Hold the rotahaler horizontally, twist barrel sharply forwards and backwards. This splits capsule into two. The capsule contents are now ready for inhalation.
5. Breathe out slowly and completely.
6. Keep rotahaler level and place the mouth piece over your tongue an dwell into your mouth. Close your lips around the mouth piece and tilt your head slightly backwards.
7. Breathe in the powder quickly and deeply as you can.
8. Hold breathe as long as you are comfortable and then remove the rotahaler from the mouth.
9. If any powder is left, repeat steps 5 to 8.
10. Open the rotahalers pulling two halves apart and discard the empty rotacap shell.
11. Reassemble the rotahaler.
12. If second dose is necessary, complete the whole process again.

It is necessary to keep the rotahaler always in its container to keep it clean. Keep it clean at least every two weeks in warm water. Dry it completely before putting them together.

The patient needs to learn the use of spacer or the rotahaler to get the maximum benefit out of such medications. They should ask their doctors or pharmacists. The children may find difficult to use inhalers or rotahalers. Spacers are of great help in such situation.

(d) Salbutamol

Salbutamol (also known as albuterol) is a bronchodilator and is useful for treating symptoms of bronchial asthma, chronic bronchitis, emphysema and other lung diseases. It works by opening up the air passages of the lungs. It relives cough, wheezing, shortness of breaths and troubled breathing by increasing the flow of air through the bronchial tubes.

Salbutamol is available as tablets, Sustained Release products, metered dose inhalers, syrups, and solution for nebulisation. The usual adult dose is 2-4 mg 3 to 4 times daily. The dose varies depending upon the product type, especially with sustained release product. One must look at the label of the product for the dosage.

Do not use without doctor's advice.

This should be used carefully in patients with cardio-vascular disorders, patients with hyperthyroidism and patients with diabetes mellitus. The tricyclic anti-depressants (like Amitriptyline hydrochloride) are to be avoided while taking this medicine as the combination may lead to serious cardio-vascular effects. The common side effects of this medicine are: nervousness or restlessness, trembling.

The guidelines for safe and effective use are:

- Do not take more than the prescribed dose. If you do not get relief after one hour of dosing, contact your doctor.
- Adhere to medication schedule. If you miss a dose, take the dose as soon as you remember. If it is time for next dose, skip the dose. Do not double your dose.
- Swallow the Sustained Release products without crushing or breaking. They are long acting products. Breaking or crushing before swallowing will destroy this technology.
- Learn the correct use of metered dose inhalers. Incorrect use would not relieve you as expected.
- Repeated use of this medicine may result in paradoxical bronchospasm. Discontinue the treatment and consult your doctor.
- Wash your mouth after every puff, if you are using inhaler with corticosteroids.

(e) Theophylline

Theophylline is a bronchodilator used to treat and/or prevent the symptoms of bronchial asthma, chronic bronchitis, and emphysema (chronic obstructive pulmonary disease). It works by opening up the bronchial tubes and increasing the flow of air through them. It is available as tablet, capsule, syrup, and extended or sustained release product.

The usual adult dose is 100-200 mg 3 to 4 times a day after food. It is also used along with corticosteroid therapy. The sustained release product when given as single dose at night would be helpful in controlling night asthma and early morning wheezing. The medicine should be used cautiously in patients with chronic obstructive pulmonary disease, cardiac failure, renal or hepatic disease, peptic ulcer, hypertension, cardiac diseases. Close monitoring of patients are often necessary when the patients are in medication with other medicines like: corticosteroids, calcium channel blockers (medicines in High Blood Pressure), erythromycin etc.

Do not use without doctor's advice.

Smoking increases the removal of theophylline and dosing adjustment may be necessary for smokers. The medicine is excreted in breast milk which may cause irritability, insomnia, or fretfulness in breast fed infant. It may be necessary either to stop breast feeding or stop the therapy. Common side effects are nausea, nervousness or restlessness. One may also experience heart burn and/or vomiting, but are not common.

The guidelines for safe and effective use of Theophylline:

- Take in empty stomach – one hour before or two hour after meal. However, you may take along with meals to reduce gastric irritation effects.
- Take extended release/sustained release/enteric coated product as it is without breaking or crushing or chewing.
- Take at regular interval as advised around the clock.

- Do not miss the dose. If you miss, take as soon as you remember. But if it is time for next dose, skip the missed dose. Do not double your dose.
- Stick to the same brand of product.
- Avoid eating or drinking large amount of caffeine containing foods or beverages such as chocolates, cocoa, tea, coffee. They may increase the stimulant effects of Theophylline in central nervous system.

(f) Corticosteroids in Asthma Care

Asthma is an inflammatory disorder with common symptoms like unproductive cough, wheezing (a fine whistling sound), chest tightness and sensation of shortness of breath. Though there is no known permanent cure for asthma, this can be adequately controlled with the use of medicines. The quality of life of the patients improves substantially. The goal of medicine therapy is to control asthma symptoms, to reduce frequency of attacks, and severity of exacerbations, and to reverse air flow obstruction. Basically there are two groups of medicines used in the management of asthma (there are other categories of medicines too): use of bronchodilators and anti-inflammatory agents. The bronchodilators cause dilation of the airways and the anti-inflammatory agents reduce the inflammation in the airways. When there is little response to bronchodilators, the anti-inflammatory agents like steroids (corticosteroids) are advised to be used to quickly regain control of asthma.

Corticosteroids are steroidal hormones produced in adrenal cortex. Inhaled corticosteroids are the most effective ant-inflammatory agents used for the treatment of persistence asthma. They are recommended for the long term control of asthma in patients using bronchodilators like salbutamol, terbutaline etc., more than once a week over a three months period and there are disturbance in sleep and activity. They block the body's inflammatory response and are the most potent form of anti-inflammatory medicines. They are very successful in preventing attacks and improving lung function. Regular use of inhaled corticosteroids reduces the risk of exacerbations of asthma.

Do not use without doctor's advice. Wash your mouth after each inhalation.

The most common inhaled corticosteroid is beclometasone. Other inhaled corticosteroids include budesonide and fluticasone. They should be used regularly to obtain maximum benefit. Symptom control is usually effective after 3 to 7 days of treatment. Long term high dose regimens of inhaled corticosteroids are used for the treatment of severe persistent asthma. Inhaled steroids reduce the need for long term use of oral corticosteroids and have less systemic side effects. The local side effects of inhaled corticosteroids include fungal infection of the mouth, dyspnoea (difficult respiration) and occasional coughing from upper airway irritation. Use of spacer reduces the incidence of fungal infection. Rinsing of mouth with water or brushing teeth after using inhaled corticosteroid is helpful in preventing fungal infection in the mouth. The coughing may be reduced by use of bronchodilators like salbutamol before using corticosteroid inhalers.

The usual dose of beclometasone using as metered dose inhaler for chronic asthma:

Adult: 200 micrograms twice daily or 100 micrograms 3 to 4 times daily.

Child: 50-100 micrograms 2 to 4 times daily or 100-200 micrograms twice daily.

The corticosteroids are also available for use through mouth as well as injection. Oral corticosteroids may be used as maximum therapy to achieve control of severe persistent asthma. Prednisolone orally or hydrocortisone as injection is used along with other asthma medicines for controlling severe asthma. As severe asthma can be fatal, prompt medical attention is very important. In order to reduce the systemic side effects, the dose should be kept minimum, the lowest dose that control symptoms.

Inhaled Corticosteroids form the first choice for preventive treatment of asthma. However, they are expensive than oral therapy. But they are not only safer but also more cost effective than oral corticosteroids on long term basis. The general guideline for using inhaled corticosteroids (beclometasone):

- It is prescription medicine and use with doctor's advice only.
- Remember it does not provide relief for acute attack of asthma. Use bronchodilators for immediate relief with doctor's advice.
- If you are using bronchodilators, use it at least 5-10 minutes before using beclometasone.
- Shake the inhaler before use. Understand the use of metered dose inhalers from your doctor or pharmacist.
- If two puffs are recommended, wait at least one minute before taking the second puff.

- Maintain the inhaler clean and unobstructed. Regularly wash it with warm water and dry it thoroughly.
- Gargle or rinse mouth with water after each use. This would prevent deposition of powders in the mouth causing fungal infection. Do not swallow this water.
- Report to your doctor if the response to therapy decreases or symptoms do not improve within three weeks. There may be need of adjustment of dose.
- Do not exceed the prescribed dose on your own. Adhere to prescribed regimen.

(g) Choice of Medicines for Asthma Treatment

The choice of drug treatment of asthma is dependent on the severity of the symptoms. If the treatment fails, this could be attributed to the lack of adherence to medication, un-controlled co-morbid conditions like allergic rhinitis, or continued exposure to tobacco smoke, air borne pollutants, or irritants.

Severity	Regimens	Comments
Intermittent	Inhaled short acting beta2 agonists [Salbutamol and Levosalbutamol]	Provides rapid relief. Adverse Effects: Paradoxical bronchospasm, tremor, tachycardia, QT interval prolongation, hyperglycemia, hypokalemia and hypomagnesemia, especially if used in high doses.
Mild Persistent	Inhaled Corticosteroids [Beclomethasone dipropionate, Budesonide, Ciclesonide, Flunisolide, Fluticasone propionate, Mometasone furoate]	Most effective long term treatment. Preferable to use the lowest dose which controls asthma. At usual dose, they are similar in efficacy. Adverse Effects: oral candidiasis (thrush), dysphonia, and reflex cough and bronchospasm. The patient is to be advised for mouth-rinsing after inhalation.
	Montelukast or Theophylline	Montelukast is less effective compared to inhaled corticosteroids. Monitoring of serum theophylline concentration may be necessary. Adverse effects are: nausea, vomiting, nervousness, headache and insomnia. At high serum concentrations, hypokalemia,

Contd....

		hyperglycemia, tachycardia, cardiac arrhythmias, tremor, neuromuscular irritability, seizures and death can occur. May interact with other drugs.
Moderate Persistent	Combination of low dose inhaled corticosteroids and long acting beta2 agonists (Salmeterol, Formoterol)	Inhaled Corticosteroids – as described above. The addition of a long acting beta2 agonist improves lung function, decreases symptoms and exacerbations. Adverse effects: tremor, hypokalemia, tachycardia and other cardiac effects.
	Combination of low-dose inhaled corticosteroids + a leukotriene modifier or theophylline	Same as described above.
Severe Persistent	Medium- or high-dose inhaled corticosteroids + a long acting beta2 agonist	Same as described above for each category of medicines.
	Medium-dose inhaled corticosteroid + a leukotriene modifier or theophylline	

CHAPTER 57

Constipation Treating Medicines

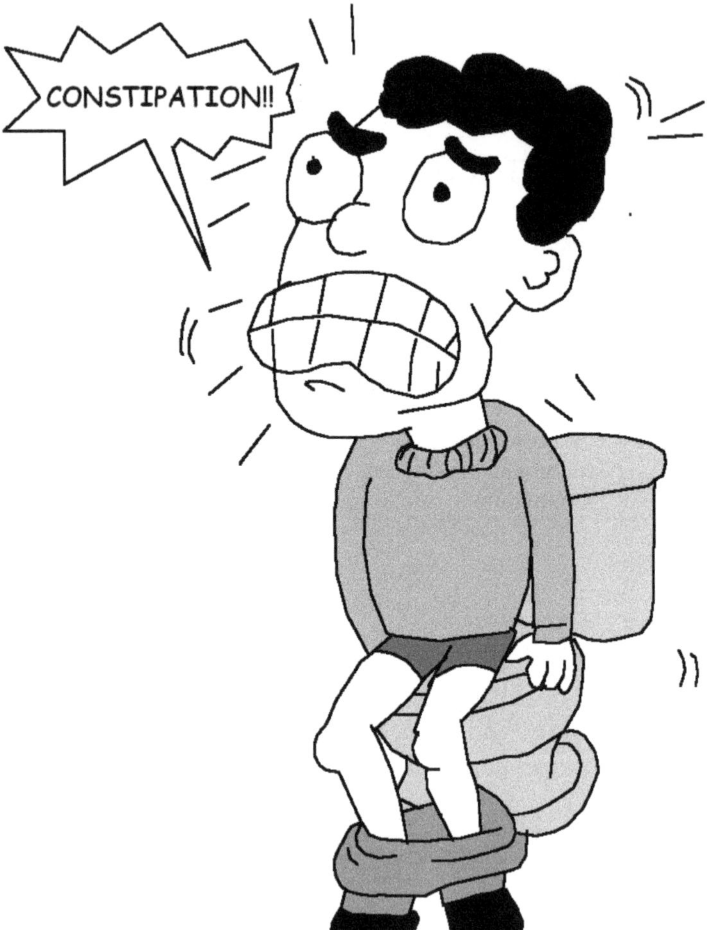

(a) Treating Constipation with Ispaghula

Constipation is often seen as frequent disturbance in quality of life and is characterized by difficult passage of hard, dry stools. The people describe this as straining to have a stool; passage of hard, dry stool; feeling of incomplete bowel evacuation. It is defined as a condition in which a person has uncomfortable or infrequent bowel movement.

There are several causes for experiencing constipation: diet, body structure, complication of child birth, a longer time for passage of intestinal contents and certain medications. It is more common in women, children and older people, though it occurs throughout the age continuum.

Acute constipation begins suddenly and noticeably. Chronic constipation may begin insidiously and persists for months or years. The frequency of bowel movements in humans generally ranges from three times a day to three times a week. In the latter case, the persons are usually symptom free. In strict sense, there is nothing like regular bowel movement.

In addition to decrease in frequency of bowel movement and difficult passage of hard dry stools, other symptoms often appear like anorexia, dull headache, lassitude, low back pain, abdominal distension, and lower abdominal distress.

Sudden development of constipation (acute) may be part of more serious illness. Consult your doctor.

Sudden development of constipation (acute) may be part of more serious illness such as acute bowel obstruction. This may be manifested by abdominal pain, vomiting and distension (bloating). Such situation needs immediate medical attention and the laxatives (medicines for treating constipation) should not be used.

The medicines available for treatment of constipation are called as laxatives or purgatives. They work by different mechanisms and accordingly classified as bulk forming, emollient, lubricant, saline, hyperosmotic, or stimulant. In the present article, use of bulk laxatives like Ispaghula is discussed.

The bulking agents add bulk to the stool. The increased bulk stimulates the natural contraction of intestine. The bulkier stools are softer and easier to pass. They act slowly and gently, the effect is usually felt from 12-24 hours but may often delay as long as 72 hours. They are known to be safe and are recommended choice for most form of constipation. Ispaghula is the most common bulk forming laxative. It is available as husk (dull white in colour) or as processed powder. The required amount of materials is mixed with a glass of water or milk. A small amount of sugar is often used to improve taste. The mixture is stirred and swallowed usually at bed time. It causes bowel evacuation next morning. The usual dose is two teaspoonful (one teaspoonful has 5 ml capacity) in glass of water or milk is given once daily at bed time. The children' dose is half to one teaspoonful given in similar way. Failure to consume sufficient fluid with bulk laxatives decreases drug efficiency and may result in intestinal or oesophageal obstruction. Other important medicines of this category include methylcellulose.

Here are few general guidelines for using bulk forming laxatives like Ispaghula and tackling constipation:

- Drink plenty of water while using bulk forming laxative. Do not swallow them dry.
- Do not use laxatives in acute and suddenly developed constipation. This condition requires immediate medical attention especially one is vomiting and has not passed even wind.
- Do not use to treat constipation associated with fever or following heart attack. One needs to be careful while treating constipation during pregnancy. Consult doctor.
- Do not use if one has problem like intestinal ulceration.
- Do not use other laxatives while using bulk forming ones.
- Do not use laxatives frequently as they may form habit.
- Consult your doctor, if treatment does not respond even after several weeks of purgative use in chronic constipation.
- Change food habits: eat high fibre diet which includes whole grain breads and cereals, raw vegetables, raw and dried fruits, and beans. Drink plenty of non alcoholic fluids (at least 6-8 glasses per day).

(b) Other Laxatives

A balanced diet, including adequate fluid in-take and fibre is of great value preventing constipation. The bowel habit varies from person to person. One can be normal even one does not have daily bowel movement as long as it causes no harm. The constipation is defined as the passage of hard stools less frequently than the one's own normal pattern. Laxatives are useful in treating constipation, but should be used when the constipation is not secondary to the underlying undiagnosed complaint. The laxatives are of value in drug induced constipation, for expulsion of parasites after anti-worm treatment and to clear the alimentary tract before surgery and radiological procedures. Prolonged treatment is rarely necessary.

Do not take other medicines within 2 hours of taking these laxatives.

The best way of treatment of constipation is food with high fibres or roughage and drinking lot of water. Eating of fruits too help. The laxatives are to be avoided within 2 hours of taking other medicines.

Three common laxatives are discussed below:

Milk of Magnesia (Magnesium Hydroxide Mixture): This is a laxative that acts by drawing more water in the gut due to osmotic gradient. This causes distension and stimulates peristalsis and bowel evacuation. It is available as suspension. It is also useful as gastric antacid but the dose is different. The medicine is contraindicated in patients with abdominal pain, nausea, vomiting or other symptoms of appendicitis, heart block, faecal impaction, rectal fissures, intestinal perforation, renal disease and patients about to deliver. It should be used with caution when the patient has rectal bleeding. The onset of action is between 30 minutes to 3 hours of taking the medicine.

The common side effects are abdominal cramping, nausea, diarrhoea and laxative dependence.

The general user guidelines:

- The usual adult dose is 2 to 4 tablespoonful at bedtime.

- Shake the bottle well before measuring the each dose.
- Drink some water each time you take a dose.
- Avoid over use to prevent laxative dependencc.
- Take plenty of fluids, diet rich in fibres and do exercise regularly.
- Do not take medicines especially which are enteric coated at the same time you take this medicine. Keep a gap of at least one hour.
- Do not take if you have diarrhoea, gut pain or dehydration.

Liquid Paraffin (Mineral Oil) Emulsion: It is useful as laxative in persons with piles who have hard and painful stools. It does not soften the stools but greases them. It lubricates the intestine. It is contraindicated in persons with abdomen pain, nausea, vomiting, other symptoms of appendicitis, acute surgical abdomen, with faecal impaction or intestinal obstruction.

It should not be used along with other stool softeners like docusate as it increases the absorption of liquid paraffin to a toxic level. The excessive use increases the possibility of loss of fat soluble vitamins (vitamin A, D, E and K). The user guidelines are:

- The usual adult dose is 1-3 teaspoonfuls by mouth at least one hour after the evening meal.
- Shake the bottle well before measuring each dose.
- Do not take with meals as it may delay gastric emptying.
- Avoid administration of other medicines together like fat soluble vitamins, anticoagulants and oral contraceptives.
- Do not use stool softeners like docusate as increased absorption of liquid paraffin may reach toxic level.
- Use under garment protection as there may be anal leakage.
- Do not use in children, pregnant or breast feeding and bedridden.

Glycerine Suppositories: The suppositories are meant for inserting into anus. They are not meant for swallowing. One suppository is to be pushed well up the anus and it is necessary to allow its stay for 15 to 30 minutes. Longer it is allowed, better it works.

After insertion into anus, it works within 30 minutes. The adverse or side effects are minimal. Some rectal reactions may occur. It draws water from intestine and forms irritant action on the mucous lining.

The user guidelines are:

- Store suppositories in refrigerator.
- Allow it to reach room temperature before use.
- Moisten with water to enhance lubrication.
- Allow the suppository to remain in anus after administration for about 15 minutes.

CHAPTER 58

Contraceptives

(a) Oral Pills

The birth control (oral contraceptives) pills are commonly known as oral pills. They contain hormones similar to Oestrogen and Progesterone, which a woman makes in her body. Most birth control pills contain both hormones: estrogen and progestin and are called combined oral pills. Oral contraceptives, which contain only progestin is known as "progestin only pills" or mini pills. These pills work by preventing the woman's ovaries from releasing an egg and making the mucous very thick at the opening of womb to prevent the entry or passage of sperm into the womb.

Combined oral pills are to be taken every day for three weeks and not to be taken for one week to allow menstruation to occur. They are available in packets of 21 or 28 tablets. In 28 tablets package, 7 tablets are dummy or iron tablets and the woman needs to take one tablet everyday without a break. This offers better user's compliance as it becomes routine to take one tablet everyday. In 21 tablets package, one tablet is to be taken everyday for 21 days and there would be a break of 7 days. A new pack is to be started after 7 days even if there is no experience of period. With either type of packs, the first tablet is to be started on the first day of the monthly period.

The mini pills (which do not contain oestrogen), though less effective than combined oral contraceptives, are better choice for breast-feeding women. These pills do not disturb the milk production like combined pills. "A pill everyday at the same time is the requirement". If taking pill is late by even few hours or forget one day's pill, it increases the chance of pregnancy.

Take the pills regularly to avoid pregnancy.

In addition to offering protection against pregnancy, these offer some additional benefits too. Some women find that taking combined oral pills help their monthly periods to be more regular with less bleeding and less pain. They too reduce the risk of ovarian cancer and pelvic inflammatory diseases in users.

The common side effects of combined pills include: irregular bleeding, nausea (sensation of vomiting) and headache. The nausea and headaches usually go after few months of use. However, if following symptoms are observed or experienced during use of combined pills, discontinue use of pills forthwith and consult your doctor:

- Severe headache with blurred vision.
- Feel weakness/numbness in arms or legs.
- Feel severe pain in your chest or shortness of breath.
- Have severe pain in the leg.
- Develop severe abdominal pain.
- Develop jaundice.

Irregular bleeding, no monthly bleeding, occasional headaches are common side effects associated with use of mini pills. The use of these pills is to be avoided in liver diseases at least till liver function backs to normal.

The efficacy of contraceptives is judged by their failure rates. The failure rate of combined pills is reported as 0.1- 8.0 % and for mini pills it is 0.5-10.0 % during the first year of use.

A small number of other medicines interact with combined oral pills and reduce the effects of the latter. The following are few examples of medicines: Rifampicin (anti TB), Barbiturates (sleeping tabs), Phenytoin (anti epilepsy), Ampicillin, Tetracycline, Cephalosporin (all antibiotics) and Griseofulvin (anti fungal). Additional protection is necessary while taking any of these medicines.

The pills are to be avoided:

✓ If confirmed or suspected pregnancy.

✓ Have breast cancer.

✓ Have abnormal bleeding.

Here below are given few general check lists for oral pill users:

- Do not miss pills. If forgets, take the pill as soon as you remember. Take the next pill at usual time even if it means taking two tablets a day.
- Inform your doctor, if you are taking other medicines.
- Do not take the combined pills if you have seizures (epilepsy), tuberculosis, hepatitis, have ever had sign of stroke, paralysis or heart disease.
- Do not use combined pills if breast-feeding.
- Do not use combined pills, if you are a heavy smoker.
- Do not change brand, without doctor's advice.

(b) Injectable Contraceptives

Family Planning (family welfare in our country) is being accepted as a human right basic to human dignity. Great progress has been made in various family planning methods and now wide choice is available for couples to select a method that best suits the individual.

Injectable contraceptive methods are the fourth most popular method worldwide after female sterilization, intrauterine device (IUD), and oral contraceptives. It has been estimated that the number of women using injectable contraceptive is more than doubled during 1995 to 2005 and more women are coming forward to use injectable contraceptives. However, the injectable contraceptives are not the part of national family welfare programme.

The most common type of injectable contraceptives is medroxyprogesterone acetate. It is progestin, a hormone similar to natural hormone the woman's body makes. It works by two ways: It stops ovulation and thickens cervical mucous making it difficult for sperm to pass through. It does not work by disrupting the existing pregnancy. There are two types of products: one meant for short term and the other for long term contraception. Both types are administered by deep intramuscular injection. The long-term products are known as depot – medroxyprogesterone acetate injection. The depot injection is required every 3 months.

There are other injectable contraceptives too. One of them is norethisterone enantate. It is progestogen and offers protection for 2 months and thus requires repetition every 2 months. Both types of these injections have lot of similarity. Women must receive full counselling from their doctors or family welfare counsellors before starting or adopting these injectable methods of contraception, concerning possible menstrual irregularities and because of prolonged activities.

The injectable contraceptives are very effective. They offer several advantages. The depot – medroxyprogesterone acetate injections can prevent pregnancy for at least 3 months, tension free life for 3 months as it does not require to have pill a day or use condom everyday, does not increase the risk of estrogen related complications like heart attack, helps preventing ectopic pregnancies (extra uterine gestation), cancer of the lining of uterus, uterine fibroids. They can be used at any age and they do not affect breast milk. Quality and quantity of milk is not harmed. Nursing mothers can use as soon as 6 weeks after childbirth.

Like other medicines, medroxyprogesterone acetate injections too have certain side effects. The common side effects include: menstrual irregularities, delayed return to fertility, reduction in bone mineral density, weight gain, depression, headache, breast tenderness, moodiness, nausea, hair loss etc. The user woman may experience light sporting or bleeding, heavy bleeding or amenorrhoea (absence of monthly period). Bleeding changes due to injectables are not harmful and it is not a sign of illness. Monthly bleeding eventually returns after injections stop.

Remember your time for next injection.

Medroxyprogesterone acetate injections should not be used during pregnancy, hormone dependent breast or genital neoplasm (tumour), undiagnosed vaginal bleeding, hepatic (liver disorders), severe arterial disease (blood pressure).

Few guidelines for safe and effective adoption of injectable contraceptives:

- Select the method of choice based on your need and appropriateness. The doctor or the health care providers will assess the products suitability for you.
- You can adopt the injectable contraceptive in the following conditions: not breast feeding a baby less than 6 weeks old, no heart disease, no blood pressure, no breast cancer, no liver disorder, not pregnant, no unusual vaginal bleeding.
- Insist on single use syringe (disposable type) to prevent spread of infection. Use of auto disable syringe is preferred. In case, they are not available, ensure that the reusable syringe and needle are properly sterilized.
- Ensure that the injections are given or administered to you following adequate hygiene and in clean area. Washing of hand with soap and water (or, use of gloves) by the injection giver is a must.

- Remember to report for next dose of injection as advised by your health care provider: every three months for depot – medroxyprogesterone acetate injection and every two months for norethisterone enantate injection. You can go to clinic up to 2 weeks early or 2 weeks late without any problem.
- The injectable contraceptives are reversible. They will not have any effect on future fertility.
- Tell your doctor that you are under injectable contraceptives. Often other medicines get affected by this.
- Immediately report your concern or unusual experience to your health care providers.

Depot DMPA

The Government of India proposes to introduce Injectable Contraceptive into the National Family Planning Programme. This is a sustained release or depot preparation of medroxyprogesterone acetate (DMPA) intended for injection once in every three months. The injection is to be given either intramuscularly or subcutaneously depending upon the preparation. The injectable contraceptive containing DMPA is known to be effective and eliminate the need of daily administration.

Because of risks of loss of bone mineral density, it is advisable to discontinue their use after two years unless the consulting gynaecologist advises continuation beyond this period.

Common side effects are: Amenorrhea, irregular bleeding, weight gain, headache, and decrease in mineral bone density.

The return of fertility can be delayed for 6 to 12 months after the last injection.

(c) Emergency Contraceptive Pills

Unwanted pregnancies are the one of the most human tragedies. They may result from unprotected sexual act, contraceptive failure, or forced sex such as rape. Sometimes couples have problems in using contraceptives because of personal reasons or lack of family planning awareness and services. This too may lead to unplanned pregnancy, which may also be unwanted. Reaction to the unwanted pregnancy may vary but it causes social, economic and emotional distress. The women may have to continue pregnancy to full term if it is not feasible to terminate or in case of feeling of guilty of requesting an abortion. A remedy for such tragedies exists.

A choice for avoiding pregnancy after an unprotected intercourse is available, called Emergency Contraceptive Pills. They are also commonly known as the morning after pills. But this is not the only option. Intra Uterine Device (IUD) is also an emergency contraception method.

The emergency pills are similar to other hormonal birth control pills. But higher doses for a short time are essential in emergency. Two regimens are available: a combination product containing ethinyl estradiol and Levonorgestrel; and single ingredient product where Levonorgestrel (a progestine like hormone) is the basic medicament. World Health Organization's Essential Drugs List prescribes Levonorgestrel in two strengths: Levonorgestrel 1.5 mg as single dose (or, two tablets of 0.75 mg strength) to be taken within 120 hours of intercourse; alternatively Levonorgestrel 750 microgram (0.75 mg) to be taken within 72 hours (3 days) of unprotected intercourse followed by 12 hours later by another tablet of same strength. This single ingredient tablets are equal to the combined products in preventing conception but are with fewer side effects and hence superior. The tablets will not work if the woman using is already pregnant. They do not induce abortion. They prevent the fertilized from attaching to the womb wall. They are only effective if used soon after having sex. These tablets prevent about 86% of pregnancy that would have occurred if no treatment had given.

Take the pills as early as possible after the unprotected sex. Sooner is taken, more effective they are.

Like other medicines this morning after pills too have some adverse effects like nausea, vomiting, headache, dizziness, breast discomfort and menstrual irregularities. But these effects are observed only in limited percentage of women using. They are reasonably safe medicines. All these days they have been made available as prescription medicines. A recent announcement by the government of India that the emergency contraceptive pills will be made over the counter medicines (OTC) (never mind there is no practical difference between a prescription and over the counter medicine as medicines of both categories are readily available for consumers without prescription) is a welcome move. They are OTC medicines in many countries. This would definitely improve the accessibility of such medicines. They would soon become popular.

In our country contraceptive use is reported to be as low as below 50 % and women resort to unsafe abortion that kill almost 20,000 annually. In such condition, the popularisation of emergency contraceptive pills definitely a welcome step. The non-prescription status along with community or public education will go in a long way improving the use of these pills for avoiding unwanted pregnancies. But the current price which is around 35 rupees is somewhat cost prohibitive. The government needs to consider and must come forward subsidizing such pills and make them available freely in all government health centres to maximise their benefits.

The success of drug therapy largely depends on the ways the medicines are used by the consumers or the patients. The success of emergency pills too is dependent on the proper use of these pills. The women need to be educated and made aware of proper use of this medicine. Here are few important tips:

- If vomiting occurs within 2-3 hours after taking tablets, take one more dose with an antiemetic medicine.
- Take pills as early as possible after the unprotected intercourse. The sooner the pill is taken more effective they are.
- Do not use during lactation.
- Use a barrier contraceptive like condoms until the next monthly period, which may be early or late.
- Consult your doctor if you develop lower abdominal pain or your next menstrual bleed is abnormally light, heavy, brief or absent.

Emergency contraceptives are less effective than regular contraceptives. They are not substitutes. Their frequent use must be avoided.

Doubling the Dose Necessary

Levonorgestrel, a progestogen, is the preferred choice for emergency contraception. The dose recommended is 1.5 mg and to be taken within 72 hours of unprotected sexual intercourse. Emergency contraceptive pills prevent pregnancy by preventing or delaying ovulation. The drug is metabolized by the cytochrome P450 enzyme system. Enzyme inducing drugs enhance this metabolism and reduce the contraceptive effects of Levonorgestrel.

Full enzyme induction can take 2 to 3 weeks to develop and similar period of time to subside after discontinuation of enzyme inducer. Anti-epileptics, anti-retrovirals, anti-TB drugs and St John's wort are potential enzyme inducers. The Committee for Medicinal Products for Human Use of European Medicine Agency has recommended doubling the dose of Levonorgestrel used for emergency hormonal contraception for women who have taken an enzyme inducer during the previous 4 weeks. 3 mg dose is suggested (two pills) when an enzyme inducer drug is taken in previous one month.

Before using, it is necessary to ensure that other drugs including herbals do not interfere with body's metabolizing system. If the woman has taken an enzyme inducer, it is reasonable to advice 3 mg of Levonorgestrel to reduce the risk of intended pregnancy. As the dose doubles just to counter the reduced efficacy of the hormone as occurs due to enzyme induction, there is no additional safety concern.

(d) Women have Better Choice

During World Population Day celebration, the Union Health Minister announced the government's strategy to introduce and promote female condoms. Indeed a good move.

Birth control is a voluntary decision of couples. In our society, women take more active part than their partners in practicing birth control or family planning. Today there are many birth control methods available to choose and use depending upon individual's need, convenience, comfort level and affordability. Reversible methods are perhaps more popular worldwide than the permanent methods of sterilization.

Though traditionally women have been using oral pills (hormones), implants, intra uterine devices (like Copper T), contraceptive sponges, spermicidal agents and female condoms worldwide, a few recently introduced methods offer significant advantages or benefits to the users. These new methods offer opportunity to the women to have more or better choice and convenience too. In the present article two important types of female contraceptives: Female Condoms (though not new, but to be introduced to the Indian women) and transdermal patches are narrated for the benefit of readers.

A female condom is a latex or polyurethane pouch that a woman or her partner needs to insert into her vagina before intercourse. Polyurethane varieties are too costly and the condoms made with less costly materials are also available in the market. Even some are in the final stages of clinical trial, a necessity for approval for mass use. In a country like ours, where even male condoms are reported to be not properly used very often leading to unintended pregnancy resulting from contraceptive failure, it is necessary that the women users need to be counselled adequately on the appropriate use of female condoms.

When used correctly the female condoms are likely to provide protection against HIV and STD (sexually transmitted diseases) like male condoms, but are reported to be less effective in practice. They are promoted as an alternative to male condoms. Here is a checklist (tips) for female condom users:

- Make sure that the condoms come with necessary supplies (usually individually wrapped condom, leaflet containing instruction and a lubricant bottle).
- Use only fresh condoms (means not opened earlier). Check the expiry date of condoms and lubricant bottle.
- Learn the techniques of using them from your family planning counsellor or other health workers.
- Do not test condoms for leaks before use as this may damage.
- Remember that they are for single use only and to be removed immediately after coitus, before you stand up.

Transdermal patches have been in practice for delivery of several types of medicines. They are sophisticated systems designed to support the passage of medicines though skin into blood, a prime necessity for medicine's action. Transdermal patches for birth control are recently introduced. They are substitutes of oral hormonal pills. At present only one patch is available in international market and some are under final stages of approval process. The patches are more convenient to use and there is no need for remembering daily use as in oral pills. One patch lasts for one week and there is no botheration for these seven days. Of course a new patch is required every week and three patches a month. For the fourth week no patch is required to allow for monthly cycle. Patch provides contraceptive effectiveness and menstrual cycle control similar to oral pills. They are substitutes of oral hormonal pills, but with added values or convenience.

You have many methods of contraception. Select the method most convenient and appropriate for you in consultation with your doctor.

The patch contains three layers: an outer protective layer, a medicated adhesive layer and a clear polyester release liner. The latter layer is to be removed just before application and on application the adhesive layer will continue to deliver the hormones to the blood stream. The patch adheres well on the skin, allowing women to perform regular daily activities such as bathing, swimming, working and exercising without interruption.

A guide for correct use of contraceptive patches:

- Apply the first patch within five days after menstruation or as per instruction given with the product.
- Change it each week for three weeks.
- Apply the patch to the new location at each time. You can apply it on the clean dry area of the skin: buttocks, lower abdomen, upper outer arm, or upper of the body but not on breasts.
- Once applied, do not remove or move to other location.
- Do not place over surface where you have applied creams, oils, and powder or make up.

There is no ideal contraceptive, which will have all merits and no demerits or risks, but the new systems offer considerable convenience and more choice to the users. There are many other systems under development and some other innovative types are already in international market. It is essential that the government should make them available through National Family Planning Programme and in the open market too to make better choice for our women as in other parts of the world. Better convenience, more acceptability.

CHAPTER 59

Cold and Cough Medicines

(a) Medicines Used in Common Cold

The common cold is an acute upper respiratory infection manifested by runny nose, watery eyes, general aches and pains, an uneasy feeling and slight fever. The nasal passages swell and the inflammation may spread to the throat. Stuffy nose, sore throat, and coughing may follow. There will be decrease in appetite. The senses of taste and smell get blocked. The common cold is also known as acute rhinitis. The symptoms appear 1 to 3 days after infection.

There are many medicines recommended to lessen the discomfort associated with the common cold. They are not meant to cure common cold. As the common cold is a virus infection, the antibiotics are of no use. Their use must be avoided. Though common cold lasts for only 4-7 days, it interferes with one's normal activities. The normal say "if treated, person feels better in one week; if not treated, person feels better in seven days." Here are few non medical self management guidelines:

- Drink plenty of fluids to prevent dehydration. Fluid intake keeps the secretions loose and easier to expel. Hot (warm) liquids will sooth a sore throat and loosen secretion.
- Gargle with warm saline. Do not drink them.
- Avoid alcoholic beverages.
- Practice frequent hand washing. As the colds are transmitted most readily by hand contact, frequent hand washing and the use of tissues are helpful preventing the occurrence.

Tea with lemon and honey, chicken soup, and hot broths are soothing and increase fluid intake.

The following categories of medicines may help: Analgesics and Antipyretics; Decongestants; and Antihistamines. They provide temporary relief. They should not be used for more than few days as rebound effect may occur. It is preferable to avoid combination medicines because such products contain several medicines which you may not need. Besides, they may have their own side effects.

Analgesics and Antipyretics: When the patient is feverish, paracetamol, aspirin, ibuprofen are effective treatment lowering fever and relieving muscle aches. Aspirin is not to be used in children and teenagers. For details see the chapter on Analgesics and Antipyretics.

Decongestants: They shrink nasal blood vessels, relieving swelling and congestion. However, they may dry out mucous membranes in the throat and make sore throat worse.

Antihistamines: They decrease nasal secretions caused by the effects of histamine. They may make you drowsy.

If the cold symptoms do not get better after few days, consult your doctor.

These medicines are often combination of several ingredients. Look at the label to prevent duplication.

Influenza is also an acute contagious viral infection with similar symptoms of common cold but is with more severe complications. Some antiviral medicines are used and vaccination is also recommended.

(b) Soothe Your Cough

The Centre for Disease Control and Prevention (CDC) of USA in its Morbidity Mortality Weekly Report dated 12 June 2007 cautioned the use of common cough and cold medicines in children under 2 years of age. It has been reported that more than 1500 children under 2 years were treated in emergency rooms across USA over doses and other adverse reactions associated with the use of cough and cold medicines in 2004 and 2005.

With monsoon setting in, many are likely to have common cold and cough. The children are more vulnerable. Cough is a symptom of diverse infections and non infection disorder. Although the cough may have several reasons but most frequently associated with common cold. Coughing is a natural reflex to lung irritation. It helps to protect the lungs against particles that have been inhaled. Coughing sometimes produces sputum – a mixture of mucous, debris and cells expelled by lungs. Cough is regarded as friend not a foe.

Basically cough is divided into two types: non productive cough and productive cough. In productive cough, also called wet cough, there is a production of sputum. The retention of sputum may impair ventilation and the lungs' ability to resist infection. A yellowish, green, or brown appearance may indicate bacterial infection. Clear, white or watery sputum does not indicate a bacterial infection but perhaps caused by virus, allergy or irritant. On the other hand, a non productive cough, also known as dry cough, serves no useful physiologic process. There is no production of sputum.

The primary objective of treatment is to reduce the number and severity of cough episodes. This would help the patients feel better during the day and sleep better at night. Cough suppressants like codeine, dextromethorphan and diphenhydramine are drugs of choice for non productive or dry cough. Codeine, a morphine derivative, reduces cough by acting centrally on the cough centres located in the medulla. The common side effects associated with cough suppressant dosage are nausea, vomiting, sedation, dizziness and constipation. In cough suppressant dosage the codeine has low toxicity and little risk of addiction. The drugs like other CNS depressants like barbiturates, sedatives, alcohol have additive CNS depression.

Dextromethorphan acts centrally on the respiratory centres in the medulla and usually recommended to suppress cough associated with allergy or common cold. Though it has wide range of safety, its overdose may cause confusion, excitation, nervousness and irritability. Respiratory depression may occur in very high doses. Additive depression of CNS occurs with alcohol, antihistamines and psychotropic medications.

Diphenhydramine is a sedating non selective antihistamine. It too acts on respiratory centres in the medulla. It is indicated to control cough that result from colds or allergy. Its side effects include drowsiness, disturbed coordination, blurred vision, respiratory depression, urinary retention, dry mouth and dry respiratory secretions. Other problems such as rotation of eye balls, contraction of neck muscles, photo allergic reactions were also reported as side effects.

In productive cough, it is not recommended to be suppressed. Treating the underlying cause like infection, fluid in the lungs, or an allergy is more important. Antibacterial therapy for infection and antihistamines for allergy are examples. Expectorants help loosen mucous by making bronchial secretion thinner and easier to cough up. Examples of expectorants are iodides, guifenesin, terpin hydrate. Mucolytics (that reduces thickness of the mucous) are recommended when thick, sticky bronchial secretions are a major problem.

Do not take cough medicines for long time without doctor's advice. Antibiotics are often of little value.

Antihistamines and decongestants are often included in cough products, even if they have no proven value. But they are useful when cough is associated with running nose and congestion. The cough medicines are available as tablets or syrups. Here are few general guidelines for using cough medicines or for managing cough:

- Do not self medicate beyond seven days. If cough does not subside, consult your doctor.
- Consult your doctor, if persistent cough is over two week duration.

- Do not use antibiotics or antibacterial agents to treat common cold or influenza. In many cases, cough is self limiting.
- Antihistamines like Chlorpheniramine maleate may cause drowsiness. Do not drive or handle heavy machineries while taking medicines with such sedating antihistamines.
- If you have asthma, or chronic obstructive pulmonary disease or congestive heart failure, do not self medicate with cough medicines. Consult your doctor.
- If your cough worsens, or you cough up blood, or develop fever, or have chest pain, or have shortness of breath, consult your doctor.
- Do not swallow water immediately after taking linctus. They should be slowly swallowed without water.
- Codeine linctus often causes addiction. One should be careful.
- Gargling with salt water, slowly dissolving throat lozenges may soothe the irritant throat and may reduce irritant cough.
- Drink plenty of fluids. Well hydrated condition may thin respiratory secretions and make them easier to cough up.
- Be careful while using these medicines for children below 2 years of age. Never use unless your doctor advises.
- Some cough medicines may interact or contraindicated in presence of certain other medicines, you must inform your doctor what medicines you are taking.
- Keep these medicines away from children.

(c) Codeine as Cough Suppressant

Codeine, chemically methyl ether of morphine, is indicated for the suppression of cough caused by chemical or mechanical respiratory tract irritation. It is a constituent of opium and its properties are similar to morphine with additional benefit being less addictive. As very small amount of codeine found in opium poppy, almost all the codeine found in modern medicines is synthesized from morphine.

Codeine is used in many medicines all around the world, usually in the form of phosphate salt or sulphate. Codeine phosphate is combined with aspirin or paracetamol for treatment of moderate to severe pain. Beside as cough suppressant, it has been also used as sedative and antispasmodic. In the 19th century it was even used as antidepressant.

As cough is very irritating, reducing cough is usually the laudable goal. The different types of cough are discussed in another chapter. The use of codeine containing cough syrup is so common that the patients often just buy them from chemists without medical consultation. Various studies suggest that the codeine cough syrups do not have much effectiveness in acute cough associated with upper respiratory tract infection or common cold, but is a powerful cough suppressant and often regarded as gold standard in cough suppression.

Cough preparations containing codeine have long been used as a substitute for heroin since it is relatively cheaper and less addictive. It acts centrally on the respiratory centres in the medulla and nucleus tractus solaris to increase the cough threshold. The codeine is well absorbed from oral intake and start acting within 15-30 minutes with 4-6 hours duration of effect. The adult dose is 10-20 mg every 4-6 hours. Reduced doses are required for very young, elderly and debilitated patients. It is not recommended for children below 2 years of age.

Do not use without doctor's advice.

Usual cough suppressant codeine dosage has low toxicity and little risk of addiction. The lethal overdose in adult is around 0.5 to 1 gram and deaths result from marked respiratory depression and cardiopulmonary collapse. The common side effects include nausea, vomiting, constipation, sedation and dizziness etc.

Codeine is contraindicated during labour when a premature birth is anticipated. Patients with asthma, chronic obstructive pulmonary disease or pre existing respiratory depression, addicted individuals should not use. The breast feeding mothers should not breast feed while taking codeine. Codeine should be used with caution if patient is simultaneously under medication with other sedatives including alcohol.

More serious problem associated with the use of codeine is addiction. Both physical and psychological dependence can develop with chronic use of codeine. However, the potential dependence is much less than that of morphine. Tolerance develops very quickly and after few weeks of regular use. Doses must be increased to produce the same effect. Upon discontinuation of use of codeine, addicts may experience withdrawal symptoms including anxiety, tremor, muscle spasm, sweating, rhinorrhea, feeling of fear etc. Though most symptoms fade fairly quickly but sleeplessness and feeling weakness may continue for some months.

These cough preparations are often abused by drug addicts and youths as alternative to strong narcotics. Some countries have banned the codeine cough preparations to avoid this misuse.

Here are the general guidelines for safe and effective use of codeine cough preparations:

- They are available usually as linctuses. They need to be sipped slowly without addition of water. These thick preparations will have smoothening effect on irritating throat.
- Look for dosage in terms of codeine amount based on the strength of the preparation. The strength is usually expressed on the label of the product as each 5 ml contains ------ mg.
- Do not use in patients with chronic obstructive pulmonary disease, patients who cannot afford inspissation of respiratory secretions and in patients who are prone to respiratory failure.
- Do not use in children below 2 years of age.
- Consult your doctor if cough persists for more than 7-10 days, if the cough becomes productive with yellow or green phlegm, develop fever or lose weight.
- Avoid alcohol or other sedating medicines while taking codeine preparations.

- May cause drowsiness and impair performance. Do not drive or handle machineries which require good attention while taking codeine products.
- Add fiber to your diet or use a stool softener if you experience constipation while taking codeine.

CHAPTER 60

Anti-Diabetic Medicines

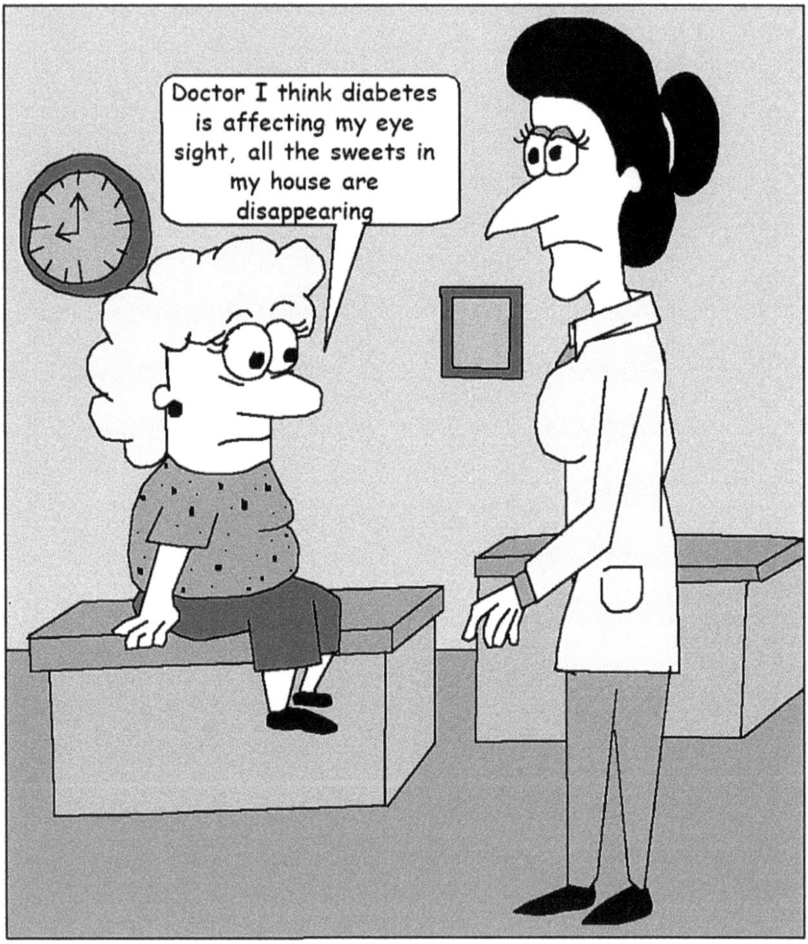
Doctor I think diabetes is affecting my eye sight, all the sweets in my house are disappearing

(a) Do's and Dont's of Insulin

One of my doctor friends comments "If you throw a stone to a crowd, it would hit a diabetic". Such is the prevalence of diabetes. It has been estimated that by the year 2025, 300 million people will have diabetes, a remarkable 5.4% of the world's projected population. India is projected to have largest number of diabetic patients by the year 2025.

In normal healthy individuals, the body's energy is met through burning of glucose (blood sugar) within the cells. The pancreas hormone, insulin, controls the passage of glucose from blood to the cells. It is also required for conversion of glucose to glycogen in the liver and formation of fatty acids in the adipose cells. Thus the lack of insulin causes an increase in blood sugar level causing hyperglycemia, a condition commonly called diabetes (diabetes mellitus). It is basically two types: type – I (insulin dependent) and type – II (non insulin dependent). Diabetes can cause serious damage to several important structures within the body. Type I diabetes treatment requires use of insulin from external source while type II can be treated with oral hypoglycemic agents and/or insulin from external source. Indeed, in type – I diabetes, the patient's survival depends on the provision of daily injections of insulin.

Insulin is a protein and would be digested before reaching the blood stream. Hence, it is not yet feasible to have oral form of insulin either as tablet, capsule or oral liquid. It is available as injection for subcutaneous administration. There are two types of insulin based on external source: animal source and human source (genetically engineered). Though both have similar efficiency in controlling blood glucose level, human insulin is more tolerable. Animal insulin often has a risk of insulin allergy, but is cheaper. There are different types of insulin preparations available in the market. These include quick acting, short acting, intermediate acting, long acting and mixed. As different types of insulin work at different speeds and for different duration, and the patients respond differently to insulin, the individual doctor decides the best insulin for his/her patient. Though injection is most common form of insulin administration, currently other modes of delivery is also available like insulin inhaler, insulin pump, etc.

Regular monitoring of blood glucose is a must for the patient under treatment with insulin. Easy to use glucometers are available. Once diet schedule and dosing of insulin is adjusted, it should be followed meticulously. Otherwise the blood glucose maintenance is disturbed. The injection of insulin subcutaneously (injected under the skin) may cause lipoatrophy, a buildup of fibrous tissue, if injection is continued at same site repeatedly. The tissue becomes spongy and avascular. The latter makes the skin anesthetized and injection is not felt. Absorption from this site becomes erratic and uncontrollable. The site of the injection must be rotated. The patients need to seek assistance from their doctors to learn the self-injection techniques.

Never change the injection schedule or meals without doctor's advice. You must take meal within 30 minutes of injection.

Like other medicines, insulin too has also side effects. The most common is lowering of blood glucose level, hypoglycemia. Serious hypoglycemia may occur with over dosing, missing of meals, inappropriate exercise, during vomiting and diarrhoea, and after drinking alcohol. The symptoms of hypoglycemia include headache, palpitations, sweating, tremor, nausea, blurred vision, increased hunger, speech and motor dysfunction etc. If hypoglycemia is suspected, blood glucose should be tested immediately and sweets, sugar or glucose be taken or given orally.

The inappropriate use of insulin can turn this life saving medicine to a dangerous drug. Here are few tips for safe and effective use of insulin injections:

- Check the dose to ensure that it is correct.
- When mixed injections are advised, draw regular insulin first and then modified insulin to the syringe.
- Allow the injection to warm up to reach room temperature prior to injection. The cold insulin injection is uncomfortable.
- Rotate the site of injection and follow all precautions used for injections like swabbing of injection site with surgical spirit.
- After injection take food within 15 minutes.

- Keep insulin in a cool place or in refrigerator. Do not freeze or allow to be exposed to high temperature like overnight in a car in winter and heat.
- If kept at room temperature, do not use after one month. Ice bags for storing insulin are available for carrying while traveling or keeping at home.
- Do not shake insulin vial. It may cause frothing and bubble formation leading to inaccuracy in dose.
- Follow regular exercise and meals as advised by your doctor. Never change the injection schedule or meals without prior consultation with your doctor.
- Always carry sugar, sweets or candy and take as you feel or suspect hypoglycemia. It can cause serious problem like brain damage if prolonged.
- Regularly monitor blood glucose level and consult your doctor, if it is not controlled.
- Do not smoke within 30 minutes of injection as smoking decreases absorption of insulin.
- Avoid alcohol.
- Never use an expired insulin product.

Finally all diabetics especially with insulin must carry an identification diabetes card. This informs others that the individual is diabetic on insulin in the event of a mishap. Research is in progress and it is not far away when the diabetic patients will have oral insulin.

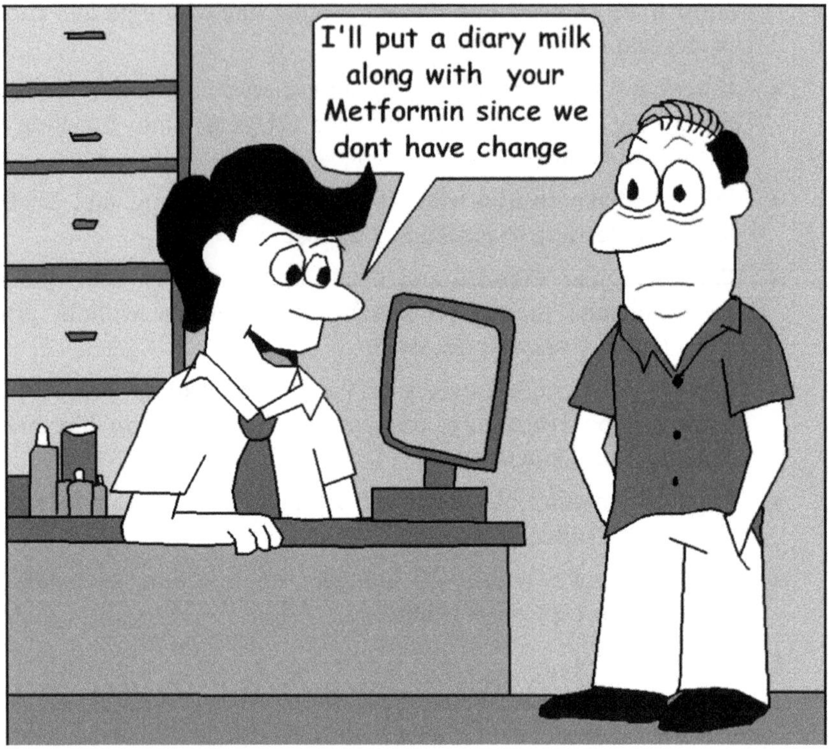
I'll put a diary milk
along with your
Metformin since we
dont have change

(b) All about Metformin

A recent article in Dutch Medical Journal reported two fatal cases of lactic acidosis resulted due to metformin use. Lactic acidosis is a rare but serious metabolic complication. The symptoms of lactic acidosis are: feeling very weak, tired, or uncomfortable; unusual muscle pain; trouble breathing; unusual or unexpected stomach discomfort; feeling cold; feeling dizzy or light headed; and sudden development of a slow or irregular heart beat. The condition is usually created by excessive accumulation of lactic acid in the blood.

Metformin is one of the popular oral anti-diabetic medicines. It is used in the treatment of type – 2 diabetes. This has been approved for use in addition to diet and exercise to control blood sugar in type – 2 diabetic patients. Chemically it is biguanide. It exerts its effect by decreasing gluconeogenesis (generation of glucose from non-sugar carbon substrates), decreasing intestinal absorption of glucose and by increasing peripheral utilization of glucose. Metformin can only act in the presence of endogenous insulin. Therefore, it is effective only in diabetics with some residual functioning pancreatic islet cells. It is useful only in treatment of type 2 diabetes, not in type 1.

The most common side effect of metformin is gastrointestinal upset, including diarrhoea, cramps, nausea and vomiting. In order to reduce gastrointestinal effects, treatment is usually initiated with a low dose which may be gradually increased. The usual recommended dose is: For ADULT and CHILD over 10 years initially 500 mg with breakfast for at least 1 week then 500 mg with breakfast and evening meal for at least 1 week, then 500 mg with breakfast, lunch and evening meal *or* 850 mg every 12 hours with or after food; usual maximum 2 g daily in divided doses.

Do not take without medical advice. Adhere to medication and meal schedule.

Metformin is just a part of a complete programme of treatment which includes diet, exercise and weight control. It is necessary to use this medicine regularly and never to stop or change the dose without your doctor's advice. The doctor may change the dose based on your sugar level control or health condition. One may be advised to have complete change of medicines if he or she becomes sick, injured, or serious infection, or need surgery. One of the major advantages of this medicine is that it does not usually cause hypoglycaemia. But even then one should be careful not to let blood sugar going too low. This may happen if one skips a meal, exercise too long, drink alcohol or under stress. The signs of low blood sugar level are: hunger, headache, confusion, irritability; drowsiness, weakness, dizziness, tremors; sweating, fast heartbeat; seizure (convulsion); fainting, comma etc.

The guidelines for safe and effective use of metformin:

- Remember the metformin is meant for treatment of type 2 diabetes only. It has no effect in type 1.
- Take the medicine as directed with respect to dose and frequency. Do not exceed the dose.
- If you miss a dose, take it as soon as you remember (be sure to take medicine with food). If it is almost time for the next dose, skip it off. Continue with usual schedule.
- If you feel you have over dosed this medicine, consult your doctor immediately. You may have symptoms of hypoglycaemia.
- Understand the signs of low blood sugar and always keep a source of sugar like candy. Use it as you experience signs of low blood glucose.
- Tell your doctor that you have kidney disease or history of heart disease. In such situation, your doctor will not prescribe this medicine.
- If you need to have an X ray or CT scan using a dye, be sure that your doctor knows that you are on metformin. You may need to temporarily stop taking this medicine.
- There are many medicines which either interfere with metformin or may cause rise blood sugar or even lower blood sugar. You must tell your doctor what other medicines you are currently taking.
- Check the label of other liquid medicines you are taking to make sure that they do not have sugar. The liquid medicines are often sugar based syrup.
- Avoid drinking alcohol while taking metformin. Alcohol lowers blood sugar and may increase the risk of lactic acidosis.
- Like other medicines, keep this out of reach of children.

(c) Glibenclamide [also known as glyburide]

This is useful for treatment of non-insulin dependent diabetes mellitus in patients who do not respond to dietary adjustment and an increase in physical exercise. It is used as supplement to the effects of diet control and exercise. This decreases blood glucose level by stimulating insulin release from functioning pancreas. This is effective if only the pancreas still continues secreting insulin. Glibenclamide belongs to sulphonyl urea group of medicines.

The common adverse effects are gastrointestinal disturbances and headache; liver disorder; hypersensitivity reactions usually in first 6-8 weeks; and hypoglycaemia particularly in elderly. The symptoms of hypoglycaemia (low blood sugar level) are: sudden severe hunger, headache, sudden anxiety, shakiness, sweating, confusion, unconsciousness and coma. Hypoglycaemia may occur if one delays or miss the schedule meal or snack, exercise much more than usual, cannot eat because of nausea and vomiting, drink a significant amount of alcohol. Patients under medications are always advised to carry some sweets like lozenges or chocolates and eat them when they experience the signs of hypoglycaemia.

Do not take without medical advice. Adhere to medication and meal schedule.

The medicine should be used with caution in elderly and patients with renal or hepatic insufficiency as there is a risk of hypoglycaemia.

Glibenclamide is available as tablet. It may occasionally lead to hypoglycaemia 4 hours or more after food. But this is usually dose related and indicates excessive dose if it occurs more frequently.

The following guidelines are suggested for safe and effective use of this medicine:

- The usual adult dose is 5 mg once a day with or immediately after breakfast. The dose may be adjusted later accordingly to the response with a maximum dose of 15 mg daily.
- Follow prescribed diet, exercise and medical regimen.
- Learn the symptoms of hypoglycaemia and take some sugar/candy/chocolate immediately as you experience of hypoglycaemia.
- Do regular monitoring of blood glucose level.
- If you miss the dose, take the missed dose as soon as you remember. But if it is time for next dose, skip the missed dose. Do not double your dose.
- Keep the medicine out of reach of children.
- Stop alcohol and smoking. Alcohol would cause unpleasant feeling like nausea, vomiting, abdominal cramps and headache. Smokers may require the higher doses of the medicine.

(d) Act Today for a Better Tomorrow: Join Diabetes Screening!

It is alarming! "India is the diabetes capital of the world. India with more than 69.2 million people with diabetes reflects every fifth diabetic is an Indian" is the reality. While type 1 diabetes cannot be prevented but type 2 diabetes is definitely preventable with life style changes. Diabetic Association of India, Mr. C. B. Wadhwa, comments "The treatment of diabetes, heart diseases and cancer is not in the hospital but in your kitchen. Nutrition is the key tool to combat the diabetes epidemic".

Diabetes is perhaps the biggest health challenge of this century. It is estimated that there would be 642 million people with diabetes globally by 2040. Of the top 10 countries in the world, India stands second with more than 69.2 million diabetics. In order to raise awareness of diabetes and related complications, the World Diabetes Day is celebrated every year on 14th November. This is the birth day of the medical scientist, Sir Frederick Banting, responsible for discovery of insulin and its use in successfully treating diabetes. The World Diabetes Day 2016 focusses on the theme "Eyes on Diabetes". It emphasizes the importance of early screening for diabetes. One of two persons with diabetes remains undiagnosed leading to the risks of complications such as disability and premature deaths.

One third of diabetics are likely to have diabetic retinopathy which may cause vision impairment and blindness. Early detection and timely treatment of diabetic retinopathy can prevent vision loss. Screening helps identifying people at sufficiently high risks which require either further investigation or direct treatment. A score involving your age, ethnicity, body mass index, waist circumference, diet, physical activities, history of high blood pressure and family history diabetes helps determining your risks. The identified high risk person must undergo oral glucose tolerance test. The test involves: overnight fasting and measurement of blood glucose level; taking 75 grams glucose and measuring blood glucose level after two hours. Though time consuming and inconvenient, it is accepted as gold standard in diabetes diagnosis. The glycocylated haemoglobin level testing is an alternative diagnostic tool but has advantage of taking blood sample at any time without the need of fasting but is expensive. These tests would decide whether the individual requires advice on life style modification or requiring treatment with medications. If the persons are at pre-diabetes stage, it is possible to prevent the progression of type 2 diabetes through life style changes. Studies have proved the possibility of reversal in glucose tolerance test to normal level with life style changes.

Diet and exercise programmes are highly effective in preventing type 2 diabetes among people who are at high risk of the disease. An intensive weight loss diet and exercise programme for 24 weeks with monthly session for two to four and half years afterwards reduces the risk of developing diabetes by more than 50 percent. This is even more effective than the common diabetic medicine, metformin. The physical activity need not be strenuous; walking is often the best form of exercise. The adoption of the following good dietary practice are helpful:

- Preferring water or unsweetened coffee or tea in place of fruit juices, soda or other forms of sweetened drinks;
- Eating at least three servings of vegetables a day including green leafy vegetables;
- Eating up to three servings of fresh fruits everyday;
- Preferring whole grain bread in place of white bread and similarly brown rice in place of white rice;
- Choosing lean cuts of white meat, poultry or sea food instead of processed meat or red meat.

People with type 2 diabetes are at greater risks from complications as the signs and symptoms of diabetes are often not felt or detected for many years and even decades. It is not uncommon to see the people first diagnosed with diabetes only after presenting with vision loss due to diabetic retinopathy or neuropathic foot wound requiring amputation. Early screening would help you manage your diabetes to have a healthier, more reproductive and longer life.

(e) Diet for Diabetic Patients

Diets have been known to have significance effects on the management of illness and promoting good health. Diet and exercise programmes are highly effective in preventing Type 2 diabetes among persons with high risk for diabetes. Life style modification (diet and exercise) should be considered as an option before starting medications in Type 2 diabetes. The basic philosophy: limit carbohydrate intake especially those coming from sugar and include protein and healthy fat. The diet plan and exercise programmes for both types of diabetes are almost same. The Type 2 diabetics may have additional goal of reducing calories and losing weight. Type 2 diabetics do not need to eat extra calories before exercise unless their blood glucose levels drops below normal.

Fruits and vegetables are high in water and fibre content and therefore low in energy density. They tend to lower postprandial glucose response. Consumption of at least three servings of whole grains per day can reduce the risk of diabetes and coronary heart diseases.

- Limit the consumption of beverages containing sugar or any caloric sweetener (including high-fructose corn syrup and sucrose) energy drinks and vitamin waters, fruit drinks, soft drinks, iced tea, and lemonade.
- Avoid processed foods which do have often added fat, sugar, and sodium. Instead, prefer high-fibre, nutrient-dense sources of carbohydrates. If on insulin, keep carbohydrate intake consistent with respect to time of day and amounts.
- Reduce salt intake (sodium).
- Eat two servings of fatty fish at least twice per week.
- Prefer liquid fats instead of saturated or trans-fat varieties, and consume leaner sources of protein (poultry, nuts, beans, and fish).

(f) Using Glucose Meters and Test Strips: Safety Tips

- **Follow instructions carefully.** Glucose meters and test strips are sold with instructions for use. You can call the manufacturer of your device or your health care provider if you have questions.
- **Ask your health care provider to watch you test yourself.** He or she can tell you if you are using your device correctly.
- **Do quality control checks of your device.** Regularly test your meter using a control solution to make sure the test strips and meter are working properly together. (Read the meter's instructions for use to see how often you should test it.)
- **Understand what the meter display means.** Be sure you know how high and low glucose values are displayed on your meter. Sometimes they are displayed as "LO" or "HI" when the glucose level is beyond the range than the meter can measure. Talk to your health care provider if you have questions.
- **Know which test site gives the most accurate results.** Readings from other areas of your body may not be as correct as fingertip readings.
    - ➢ Readings from alternate sites—such as your forearm or palm—can be less accurate than fingertip readings when your glucose levels change quickly (like after you eat or during exercise).
    - ➢ Take a reading from a fingertip if you think your blood glucose is low, if you don't normally have symptoms when your blood glucose is low, or if results from an alternate test site don't match how you feel.
- **Know when and how to clean and disinfect your glucose meter.** Cleaning and disinfection instructions can vary, so always read and follow the directions in your manual.
- **Know when to report device problems.**

[https://www.fda.gov/ForConsumers/ConsumerUpdates/ucm049051.htm?source=govdelivery&utm_medium=email&utm_source=govdelivery; Accessed on 16 May 2017*]*

CHAPTER 61

Anti-diarrhoeal Medicines

(a) Fighting Cholera

The recent outbreak of cholera in few districts of Orissa was a serious concern in public health. It has been reported more than 100 people died of the cholera. Similar outbreak was also reported recently in two northern province of Iraq. Though cholera has been rare in industrialized nations, it continues to be the problem of other parts of the world including India.

Cholera is an acute diarrhoeal illness caused by the bacterium *Vibrio cholerae*. Within less than 1 day to five days of infection, the patients develop copious, painless watery diarrhoea (also called rice water stools) often with vomiting leading to severe dehydration. If not promptly treated, it leads to deaths. Several strains of cholera bacterium have been identified.

Cholera infection is associated with poor sanitation and a person gets cholera by drinking water or eating food contaminated with cholera bacterium. In an epidemic, the source of contamination is usually the faeces of infected person. Cholera bacteria produce a toxin that causes the small intestine to secrete immense amounts of fluid rich in salts and minerals. The resulting critical water and salt loss leads to severe dehydration. The dehydration is manifested by intense thirst, muscle cramps, weakness and minimum urine production. The eyes become sunken and the skin looses elasticity. Severe dehydration can develop quickly. The loss of fluids and minerals from the body is the main cause of deaths.

Treatment consists mainly of oral or injectable rehydration. Most of the cases, adequate Oral Rehydration Salts (ORS) may be sufficient to prevent and treat dehydration. ORS contains glucose, sodium chloride, potassium chloride, and sodium citrate. ORS packets are available free from government hospitals, and are also supplied though Anganwadi centres. ORS for use must be prepared by dissolving the contents of the pack in required quantity of boiled and cooled drinking water. The amount of water to be used depends on the pack size of ORS. This is written on the label of the pack. Too concentrated solution may be dangerous. The use of ORS is recommended even if the patient vomits. It is not that all the drink will be vomited. However, the critical patients need to be treated with intravenous fluids in health facilities.

ORS is a live saving medicine. Do not use prepared ORS (drink) after 24 hours.

Antibacterial drugs (antibiotics) may shorten the course of infection and diminish the severity of illness, but rehydration therapy is most important. Tetracycline is the usual antibiotics of choice, but resistance to it are increasing. Other antibacterial medicines which may be helpful include co-trimoxazole, erythromycin, doxycycline, furazolidine, chloramphenicol etc., if the organism is sensitive. The usual adult dose of tetracycline is 250-500 mg four times a day (every six hour one dose). The treatment period is around 3-5 days. Tetracycline should not be used in pregnant women or children under 8 years of age, as it is known to cause damage or stain baby's teeth and bones. Milk, gastric antacids, products containing milk like tea, coffee, ice cream etc., affect the functioning of tetracycline (absorption is reduced). Hence, it is recommended that these foods should not be taken one hour before or after the medication. The tetracycline decomposes into toxic product and it is dangerous to use expired medicines.

Vaccines are helpful in providing protection for several months against cholera.

Vibrio cholera 01 strain can survive on a variety of foods even up to 5 days in normal condition and up to 10 days at refrigerated condition. The acidic and dried foods are usually safe as in acidic condition is organism will not survive. Gamma irradiation and cooking at temperature above 70 °C destroy this cholera bacterium.

Here are few guidelines for prevention and fighting cholera:

- Dispose of the human faeces hygienically.
- Use safe drinking water. Boiled and cooled water or water treated with chlorine and iodine is safe. Tea and Coffee as they are prepared with boiled water are safe.
- Maintain good food hygiene: Ensure thorough cooking and eat while the foods are still hot. Avoid under cooked or raw fish. Prevent cooked food being contaminated with raw foods, water, ice etc. Avoid raw fruits and vegetables unless they are freshly peeled by you. Avoid salads. Avoid outside foods and beverages especially from street vendors.
- Use ORS to prevent dehydration and restore hydration, even if one is vomiting. Follow the guideline given on the label to prepare ORS for use using boiled and cooled drinking water. Throw the unused solution after 24 hours of preparation, if left excess.
- Use antibiotics only after medical consultation.
- If the patient looks serious, transfer him or her immediately to the health facility.
- If you suspect of cholera, immediately inform to the nearest health centre.

(b) Oral Rehydration Salts

Dehydration coupled with under nourishment is the main reason of death in diarrhoea. Oral Rehydration Salts (ORS) is recommended as first line of treatment. The introduction of ORS in 1971 has revolutionized the treatment of watery diarrhoea and reducing fatalities all over the world. While introducing the new ORS formula the World Health organization has said, "This will save millions of lives and will reduce the severity of diarrhoea and vomiting, the number of hospitalisations, the need for costly intravenous fluid treatment and the length of illness".

The current formula:

Sodium Chloride	– 2.6 g
Glucose, anhydrous	– 13.5 g
Potassium Chloride	– 1.5 g
Trisodium citrate, dihydrate	– 2.9 g

For dissolving in one litre of freshly boiled and cooled drinking water.

When glucose and trisodium citrate are not available, they may be substituted by 27 g sucrose (common sugar) and sodium bicarbonate 2.5 g respectively for one litre solution.

Increased thirst, restlessness, irritability, decreased skin turgor, dry mouth and tongue, absence of tears and sunken eyes are few common signs of dehydration. ORS is a safe, effective and practical maintenance therapy in dehydration. Oral glucose enhances the intestinal absorption (entry into blood) of salt and water and thus corrects the electrolyte and water deficit. The new formula of ORS with reduced concentration of sodium and glucose is more effective and reduces the need of intravenous fluids.

The dose is 200-400 ml solution for adult after every loose motion and for infant and child quantity of fluid is based on degree of dehydration. In case of vomiting, it may be discontinued for 10 minutes and then rate of giving the oral solution should be reduced.

The common adverse effects include vomiting - perhaps indicating too rapid administration; excessive sodium and excessive potassium in blood may result from over dose in renal impairment or administration of too concentrated solutions.

The ORS packets are usually available free at all primary health centers, sub centers and hospitals. They are free supplied through Anganwadi centers too in village area. If a WHO formula is not available, a homemade ORS can be used until the proper ORS is obtained. The earlier the treatment provided the better it is for the patient. The homemade ORS can be made by taking one pinch of common salt (three finger) and 1 scoop of sugar (four finger) for dissolving in one glass (200 ml) of freshly boiled and cooled drinking water. Before adding sugar, the taste of the drink to be confirmed that it is less salty than tears.

Important things to remember while using ORS:

- ORS treatment does not reduce frequency of stools.
- It only prevents dehydration, the major cause of death in acute diarrhoea. Immediately consult doctor if condition looks to be serious.
- ORS sachets should be reconstituted as with recommended quantity of freshly boiled and cooled drinking water. The different sachets may have different quantity of powders.
- Once prepared it should be used within 24 hours of preparation. Throw out the excess remaining.

Quantity of water (mentioned in the packet for dissolving ORS powder) is important to have the correct Osmolarity for water absorption and thus prevent dehydration, the main reason for deaths. Often people overlook this aspects believing concentrated solutions are better as patients sometimes refuse to take ORS solutions.

(c) ORS with Zinc – an Effective Treatment for Paediatric Diarrhoea

The latest United Nations Children' Fund (UNICEF) report says "5000 kids die daily under the age of five in India". An alarming figure despite several initiatives and rapid progress in medical and related health sciences! The more painful is that this happens mainly due to preventable causes. Among the various causes, diarrhoea is the most important reason which accounts for nearly 10-20% of deaths.

Diarrhoea is having loose or watery stools at least three times per day, or more frequently than normal for an individual. Diarrhoea is a common symptom of gastrointestinal infections caused by a wide range of pathogens, including bacteria, viruses and protozoa. Rotavirus is the leading cause of acute diarrhoea, and is responsible for about 40 per cent of all hospital admissions due to diarrhoea among children under five worldwide. Though most episodes of childhood diarrhoea are mild, acute cases can lead to significant fluid loss and dehydration, which may result in death or other severe consequences if fluids are not replaced at the first sign of diarrhoea.

In normal condition the body takes up water and salts through drinks and food & looses them through stool, urine and sweat. The balance is maintained as the water and salts pass back from bowel to the blood. In case of diarrhoea, the bowel does not work in natural way. The more loss of water and salts occur than less absorption of them from bowel. This leads to larger than normal loss of water and salts causing dehydration. There are other reasons too for dehydration of children during diarrhoea. Water constitutes the greater proportion of body weight in children than adults. Young children use more water over the course of the day because of high metabolic rate and their kidneys are less able to conserve water compared to older children and adults. Dehydration can also occur due to vomiting which often accompanies diarrhoea.

Irrespective of cause of diarrhoea, loss of large quantity of water and electrolytes causing dehydration is the main factor responsible for deaths in acute diarrhoea. Hence the management of acute diarrhoea is aimed to prevent dehydration and supplement electrolytes. The International Centre for Diarrhoeal Disease Research, Bangladesh, has been advocating the use of Oral Re-hydration Therapy (ORT) since 1970s with the Oral Re-hydration Salts (ORS). When the ORS solution reaches the small intestine, the sodium and the glucose in the mixture are transported together across the lining of the intestine. The sodium which is now in higher concentration in the intestine, promotes water absorption back into the body from the bowel. (The pathogens responsible for causing diarrhoea damage the intestine causing excessive loss of water and electrolytes than the absorption). The discovery that the sodium and glucose are transported together across the small intestine led to the discovery of ORS. Further research on use of ORS led to development of new formula of ORS. The new formula is known as low osmolarity ORS. The new formula is shown to have additional clinical benefits like decreased stool output and vomiting in addition to preventing dehydration like old ORS. WHO and UNICEF have been recommending the use of new low osmolarity ORS.

Sodium Chloride	–	2.6 g
Sodium Citrate	–	2.9 g
Potassium Chloride	–	1.5 g
Glucose (anhydrous)	–	13. 5 g

The whole quantity is to be dissolved in one litre of recently boiled and cooled water.

It is important to realise that accurate weighing and thorough mixing and dissolution of ingredients in the correct volume of drinking water is important. Administration of more concentrated solution can result in hypernatraemia. ORS is recommended for both children and adults.

Zinc not only reduces the severity of childhood diarrhoea but also improves immunity of the child.

A recent development in diarrhoeal treatment is addition of Zinc to the ORS regimen. Zinc is an important micronutrient for child's overall health and development. Zinc is lost in greater quantities during diarrhoea. Replacing the lost Zinc help the child recovers and keeps the child healthy in the coming months. The research confirmed that Zinc supplementation given during an episode of diarrhoea reduces the duration and severity of the episode. It lowers the incidence of diarrhoea too in the following 2-3 months. It improves appetite and growth. Zinc increases the ORS uptake and reduces the inappropriate drug use with antibiotics and anti-diarrhoeal medications. Realizing the importance of Zinc in the management of childhood diarrhoea, the Government of India too revised its diarrhoeal treatment guidelines and introduced Zinc supplementation. The new guideline recommends the use of 20 mg zinc sulphate dispersible tablets. Dose for children aged between 2 months to 6 months is half tablet (10 mg) while the dose for older children is 1 tablet a day. The tablet is to be dissolved either in breast milk or drinking water before giving to children. It is advised that the child be given the Zinc for 14 days beginning from the day diarrhoea starts.

Though there are other drugs like antibiotics and anti-motility agents are often used, none of them have convincing evidence to be effectively stop diarrhoea and safe. Antibiotics are not effective against most diarrhoea causing organisms. Anti-motility drugs though temporarily reduce cramps and pain, but delay elimination of causative organisms and may prolong illness. They are harmful especially in children below five years of age. The current WHO Model Formulary (2008) lists only ORS and Zinc as medicines for diarrhoea in children.

The WHO suggests that acute diarrhoea in children should always be treated with ORS according to plan A, B and C. The plan A, B and C is based on degree of dehydration.

Plan (Degree of Dehydration)	**Management Plan**
Plan A (No dehydration)	Nutritional Advice, Increased fluid intake (ORS, soup, rice, water and yoghurt, or even water) and zinc supplementation. Continuing feeding especially breast milk is encouraged. Parents should be advised about the circumstances in which they should seek medical advice.
Plan B (Moderate dehydration)	4 hour treatment plan. 75 ml/kg body weight of oral re-hydration solution over 4 hour period. A larger amount of solution can be given if the child is continued to have frequent stools. In case of vomiting, re-hydration must be discontinued for 10 minutes and then resumed at a slower rate. Breast feeding on demand; for others milk and nutritious food after completing 4 hours of re-hydration. Zinc supplementation as soon as child can eat and completed 4 hours of re-hydration. Re-assess the status of the child after 4 hours. ORS is to be continued, even if the dehydration is controlled, as long as the child continues to have diarrhoea.
Plan C (Severe Dehydration)	Hospitalization is necessary. Priority is to start re-hydration.

In addition to continuing feeding, the effective treatment plan for childhood diarrhoea includes the use of ORS and Zinc. Though Zinc is not a prescription drug, its availability is not easy in retail pharmacy. ORS is readily available and often they are flavoured. The flavoured ORS are preferred by children. The combined use of new ORS and Zinc is proved to be more effective than simple new ORS. If a strategy is designed to develop a combo pack containing both, the regimen would be more popular and can be effectively used in controlling childhood diarrhoea which would go in a long way in reducing diarrhoeal related deaths in children.

(d) Zinc in Diarrhoea

Diarrhoea continues to be one of the leading causes of deaths among children. The use of Oral Rehydration Therapy using ORS has dramatically decreased mortality from diarrhoeal deaths. But it does not decrease the duration or severity of diarrhoea episode. Recent evidence showed that zinc supplementation (in addition to ORS) significantly reduces duration and severity of an episode of diarrhoea.

Zinc is an essential micronutrient and has multiple physiological and metabolic functions such as physical growth, development and maintenance of healthy immune system etc. The major source of zinc intake is through diet, especially meat. Though it is difficult to assess individual zinc deficiency, it is estimated that around 21 percent of population around the world are at risk of zinc deficiency. It has been well recognized that the zinc deficiency is one of the major risks to child health. It is linked to diarrhoea, lower respiratory tract infection and malaria.

Use of up to 20 mg zinc for 14 days is well tolerated and does not produce significant adverse reactions. The most common side effects are nausea and vomiting. There is a risk of copper deficiency in case of excess zinc intake. But at the recommended dose it has no effect on copper status. The use of zinc in renal failure requires caution as it gets accumulated. It interacts with some common drugs like iron, ciprofloxacin, calcium salts, ofloxacin etc. While with other medications, it is preferable to consult doctor for advice.

Zinc not only reduces the severity of childhood diarrhoea but also improves immunity of the child.

Zinc is supplied as zinc sulphate. It is available as dispersible tablets or as syrup. The tablets are cheaper. The dispersible tablets can be dispersed in breast milk, in oral rehydration solution or in water on a small spoon before giving to children to swallow. The older children may chew tablets or swallow them with water. The Government of India has made arrangements to make the zinc tablets available along with ORS in all health facilities percolating even to the level of Anganwadi centre. As zinc is a non prescription drug, people have no problem in purchasing it too.

Zinc supplementation is recommended in addition to Rehydration Therapy with ORS. It is not meant to replace ORS or any other drug treatment. ORS remains the safe and effective therapy for fighting dehydration, major reason of mortality. Zinc supplements given during an episode of acute diarrhoea not only reduce the severity and duration of the episode; if given for 14 days zinc also reduces the incidence of new episodes of diarrhoea in the 2 to 3 months following treatment.

General Guidelines:

- Remember the zinc supplementation is in addition to giving ORS to children during diarrhoea.
- Dose: for children between 2-6 months: 10 mg (Half tablet) per day dissolved in breast milk. For children above 6 months: 20 mg (one tablet) per day either dissolved in breast milk or drinking water.
- The duration of treatment with zinc is 14 days. It needs to be continued for the full course even if your child recovers from diarrhoea.
- Tablets are available as dispersible one. It can be dispersed in a spoon of breast milk or water before giving to the child. Syrups are costlier than tablets.

CHAPTER 62

Medicines for Filariasis

The very sight of unusual swollen legs is frightening. A dreadful but is preventable condition. This is Filariasis, commonly known as Elephantiasis, is a threadworm infection. Lymphatic Filariasis affects 120 million people living in 83 countries with India accounting for 40% of the global prevalence of infection. The disease has been prevalent since antiquity. There are around 473 million people are exposed to the risk of bancroftian infection; of these about 125 million in urban areas and about 348 million in rural areas. Over 23 million suffer from filarial disease manifestations.

Filariasis has been one of the major public health problems in the country. The disease is endemic in several states of the country: Andhra Pradesh, Assam, Bihar, Chhattisgarh, Goa, Gujarat, Jharkhand, Karnataka, Kerala, Madhya Pradesh, Maharashtra, Orissa, Uttar Pradesh, West Bengal, Pondicherry, and Tamil Nadu. Filaria is a long, thread like roundworm called *Wuchereria bancrofti* that lives as a parasite in the body of human beings and animals. When a mosquito bites an infected person, it takes up the larvae with the blood. These larvae develop in the mosquito. When this mosquito bites again to another person, larvae enter the new person and infect him. The adult worms live in the lymph (a fluid) of the infected person. The worm blocks the flow of the lymph and cause severe swelling of legs, causing elephantiasis. It can affect breast or scrotum. This swelling of leg makes the person ugly and frightening. The infection is also caused by *Brugia malayi*.

The government of India in its health policy fixes the goal to free the country from lymphatic Filariasis by 2015. In order to address the issue, the government of India launched Mass Drug Administration programme for administering single dose of Diethylcarbamazine citrate (DEC). DEC is available as 50 mg and 100 mg tablet. The recommended dose:

Age in years	Number of tablets (100 mg)
2 - 5 years	One tablet
6 -14 years	Two tablets
15 years and above	Three tablets

The government declares one day of the year as National Filaria Day and this year it was November 15 when MDA was promoted. Some states have not yet completed this MDA programme and they would be completing before the end of the year. The single dose administration of DEC tablet(s) is recommended to all individuals in the area; however, it should not be given to children below 2 years, pregnant, and seriously ill persons. The government has even implemented the fortification of common slat with DEC in some areas of the country.

Complete the course of treatment.

The use of DEC is associated with side effects like mild fever, headache, giddiness, aches, vomiting etc., especially in persons who have microfilaria in their blood. But these symptoms are mild and will disappear within a day or so.

In order to give further boost to the filaria control programme, it is now intended to use a combination single dose therapy with Albendazole. This is proposed to be initiated as MDA in all endemic districts during 2008. The revised dosage schedule is:

Age in years	Number of tablets (100 mg) of DEC	Number of Albendazole tablets (400 mg)
2-5 years	One tablet	One tablet
6-14 years	Two tablets	One tablet
15 years and above	Three tablets	One tablet

Albendazole has additional benefits as it makes the intestine free from worms. They should be administered or taken after the meals but not on empty stomach as they may cause stomach upset. This will kill the microfilaria present in individuals and thus mosquitoes will no longer be able to spread the disease. This combination therapy is recommended for once a year for 5 to 7 years to completely make the community free from infected persons and the future from lymphatic Filariasis.

Here are few general guidelines for safe and effective use of DEC alone and also in combination with Albendazole in making our country free from the disfiguring and dreadful Lymphatic Filariasis:

- Consume DEC tablets alone or in combination with Albendazole in recommended dose preferably on National Filaria Day when MDA is campaigned.
- Swallow the tablets with plenty of water only after food. Do not take on empty stomach.
- Do not use in children below 2 years of age, pregnant women and in seriously ill persons.
- You may experience self limiting side effects like mild fever, body aches, nausea, vomiting etc., if you are infected. If these symptoms do not disappear, consult your doctor or health professional.

As the disease is spread by mosquitoes, protect yourself and family members from mosquito bites. And also avoid water collection in and around the house to prevent mosquito breeding.

CHAPTER 63

Medicines for Anaemia

(a) Iron in Anaemia

Anaemia is a common health problem in our country. It has been reported that 9 out of 10 adolescents, children and pregnant women are anaemic. This is responsible for 40% of 100000 maternal deaths that occur every year due to complications of pregnancy and childbirth. Of the various types of anaemia, iron deficiency anaemia is most common.

Iron deficiency anaemia is diagnosed by estimating the haemoglobin level in blood. Haemoglobin transports oxygen to the tissues. The body requires a good supply of oxygen for proper functioning. Iron is a component used by bone marrow to produce haemoglobin. Thus the deficiency of iron in the body causes anaemia. The normal haemoglobin level is 11-13 gram percent or gram per dl (decilitre). It is further divided for classifying anaemia during pregnancy as: mild 10-11 g%, moderate 7-10 g% and severe less than 7 g%. Iron deficiency anaemia is caused by menstrual iron loss, any slow but chronic loss of blood, iron poor diet. This also occurs during and after pregnancy because of expanding blood volume of mother, demand of foetus and placenta, blood loss during childbirth. The repeated pregnancy depletes the body's stores of iron leading to anaemia. Patients who suffer from bleeding piles, stomach ulcers or hookworm infestation also may suffer. The common symptoms of anaemia are weakness, exhaustion, lassitude (faintness), anorexia (lack of appetite), glossittis (tongue irritation) and stomatitis (inflammation of mouth). In severe cases it is reflected by palpitation, dyspnoea (difficulty in breathing), oedema and cardiac failure. Iron deficiency is also associated with behavioural or learning problem in children.

The total iron content in the human body is approximately 50 mg/kg in men and 37 mg/kg in women. Approximately 67% of body's iron is in haemoglobin. The iron deficiency can also be tested by measuring iron level in the blood.

Iron deficiency anaemia can be treated with iron preparations. "Though various types of iron preparations are available in the market, many of them are irrational and undesirable" says a study conducted by Drug Action Forum – Karnataka. The use of these products increases the cost of therapy, the study report comments. Oral form of iron is preferable. The injectable irons are not only dangerous but are costly too. The following ferrous form of iron are mentioned in WHO's formulary: ferrous sulphate, ferrous fumarate and ferrous gluconate. They differ marginally in efficiency and the choice is usually decided by incidence of adverse effects and cost. The ferrous sulphate preparations are cheapest. The oral dose of elemental iron for treatment of iron deficiency anaemia in adults is 100-200 mg daily with meals. The recommended preventive dose in high-risk women is 60 mg elemental iron daily. The approximate elemental iron content of various iron salts: ferrous sulphate 300 mg (60 mg iron), dried ferrous sulphate 200 mg (65 mg iron), ferrous fumarate 200 mg (65 mg iron) and ferrous gluconate 300 mg (35 mg). Sustained release iron preparations (tablets or capsules) are expensive but have fewer symptoms of gastric irritations.

Take iron preparations after food to reduce gastric side effects. Keep away from reach of children.

Constipation, diarrhoea, dark stools, nausea, epigastric pain, and gastrointestinal irritation are common adverse effects associated with iron therapy. If adverse effects arise with one salt, dosage can be reduced or change made to an alternative iron salt. Ferrous sulphate tablets are usually sugar coated. The children may find them as colourful candy. The medicines must be kept out of reach of children. The toxic ingestion of iron can be fatal.

Here are few guidelines for using iron preparations in treating iron deficiency anaemia:

- Use iron preparations only if diagnosed as iron deficiency anaemia or use in prophylaxis in poor diet condition and pregnancy.

- Ferrous salts are preferable: like ferrous sulphate or ferrous fumarate. Tablets are preferable than other forms.
- Take iron preparations after food (meal) to reduce gastric irritation.
- Do not eat cheese, yogurt, eggs, milk, spinach, tea, or coffee etc., within 1 to 2 hours of taking iron.
- Drink liquid iron preparations after mixing with water and through a straw to prevent staining of teeth. At least rinse mouth with water after swallowing.
- Taking iron causes black stool and do not worry for this. If you experience constipation, use stool softener.
- Iron preparations may affect action of other medicines. Tell your doctor that you are taking this. Do not self medicate long time with iron preparations without your doctor's advice.
- Keep away from children. The children may mistake iron tablets as candy. Poisoning can be fatal.

(b) Folic Acid Preventing Birth Defects

Neural Tube Defects (NTDs) is one of the common and serious birth defects. Each year 3-4 lakh infants worldwide are born with NTDs. The incidence of NTDs in general population varies from 1 per 1000 pregnancies in USA to as high as 12 per thousand in some communities in India. NTDs are birth defects of brain and spinal chord. This results in either some paralysis of legs or still born or death shortly after birth. But there is enough evidence that folic acid supplementation before conception and during pregnancy significantly reduce the risk of NTDs.

Folic acid is a member of Vitamin B group. It is essential for the synthesis of DNA (Genetic Code) and cell division and development. The requirements of folic acid are related to metabolic rate and cell turn over. There is increased need of folic acid during pregnancy, lactation, and infancy, haemolytic anaemia and blood loss etc. The deficiency of folic acid results in impaired cell division and protein synthesis. The function of folic acid is closely related to that of vitamin B_{12} (cyanocobalamin). In fact they work interdependently. A deficiency of either of these vitamins results in a serious anaemia. The folic deficiency can occur as a consequence of vitamin B_{12} deficiency.

The deficiency symptoms of folic acid include paleness, weakness, irritability and forgetfulness, reduced acid secretion in the stomach and nerve damage. The most common laboratory feature is megaloblastic anaemia. This type of anaemia is characterized by large RBCs circulating in the blood. As vitamin B_{12} is essential for the metabolism of folate, a megaloblastic anaemia responsive to folic acid administration is a feature of pernicious anaemia. Folic acid administration in pernicious anaemia may correct the anaemia but not the other problems associated with pernicious anaemia. Folic acid thus masks the symptoms of pernicious anaemia, caused by Vitamin B_{12} deficiency without giving real benefits. Hence the high dose products of folic acid should be used only with doctor's advice failing which the diagnosis pernicious anaemia will be difficult.

You must take Iron and Folic Acid tablets during pregnancy as advised by doctor or health worker.

The dietary source of folic acid is fresh leafy vegetables, fruits, liver and other organ meats, dried yeasts. Cooking destroys this vitamin. Body stores only a small amount in the liver, a diet lacking in folic acid leads to a deficiency within a few months. Deficiency may occur in pregnant women on diets that lack green leafy vegetables and legumes. Infants too develop deficiency when folic acid content of their formula is low. People who have diseases of small intestine may have trouble absorbing folic acid. Certain anti-epileptic drugs and oral contraceptives decrease the absorption (entry into blood) of this vitamin. Alcohol interferes with the absorption and metabolism of folic acid. Those who drink large amount of alcohol may also develop deficiency.

Though folic acid toxicity is virtually nonexistent, it may increase the frequency of seizure in epileptics and worsen the neurologic damage in people who have vitamin B_{12} deficiency in doses of 100 times the recommended daily dose.

The guidelines for safe and effective use of folic acid:

- Use folic acid with doctor's advice only.
- Donot use in undiagnosed anaemia as it may mask the Vitamin B_{12} deficiency anaemia. Vitamin B_{12} deficiency needs to be excluded before starting treatment with folic acid for anaemia.
- 400 microgram (1000 microgram makes 1 milligram) folic acid per day by pregnant women (prior to 1 month of conception to 3 months after conception) is recommended to prevent neural tube defects.
- 5 mg folic daily is recommended for pregnant women who have previously had a baby with NTD or have diabetes, or under anticonvulsant (for epilepsy) treatment.
- Inform your doctor, if you are taking other medicines as many medicines interact with folic acid.

CHAPTER 64

Vaccines

(a) Immunization - Saving Children through Vaccination

The millions of children die every year due to six dreaded but preventable diseases: Diphtheria, Whooping Cough, Tetanus, Polio, Measles and Tuberculosis. Vaccination is proved to be the best strategy to fight against these diseases to reduce mortality. The proportion of infants (less than one year of age) reaching their first birthday who were fully immunized according to our immunization policy was just 49% in 2001. Since then, many strategies have been adopted to cover more children under the programme and the government of India set a target to eradicate polio from this country by the year 2005. Though we failed to achieve the target in stipulated time, now the country has achieved a distinction of no polio case in 2011. This success story is due to persistence all out effort of universal immunization.

Vaccination (also called immunization) is perhaps the most important development in modern medicine in fighting diseases and reducing mortality. Edward Jenner was the first physician to discover the benefits of vaccination. He overheard a dairymaid saying that she could not catch small box since she had already had cowpox, a relatively milder disease. He experimented the principle and gifted the benefits of vaccination to the world. This is the genesis of vaccination.

Vaccines are the medicinal products used to develop resistance artificially (immunity) against infectious diseases. They contain noninfectious parts of bacteria or virus or whole organism that have been altered so that they cannot cause diseases. On receipt of the vaccine, the body develops immune defenses (antibodies). These formed antibodies protect the individual when he/she subsequently gets exposed to the corresponding infectious bacteria or virus. But this protection is very specific. Polio vaccine can protect against polio only. Tetanus vaccine protects against tetanus only and so on. We need to get immunized or vaccinated against the disease(s) we intend to protect ourselves. Despite of tremendous development in the field of science, technology and medicine, we still do not have vaccines against many killer diseases including HIV/AIDS. But efforts are on.

Vaccines are one of the most important public health interventions. Immunize your children to protect them from killer diseases. India has been declared free of polio.

Vaccines available today are highly reliable and most people tolerate them well. But however, occasionally they cause some side effects. Some vaccines cause local reactions at the site of injection like swelling, pain, redness, tenderness or development of sterile abscess. In such cases, the doctor or health worker should be consulted. Use of un-sterilized syringes or needles carries risk of transmission of hepatitis B and HIV. Fortunately government now proposes to use auto-destructible syringes during vaccination there by making injection practices much safer.

Government of India under universal immunization programme intends to cover all children for vaccination against the above six killer diseases. The five vaccines: tetanus, diphtheria, whooping cough (pertussis), measles and tuberculosis (BCG) are administered as injections while polio vaccine is given orally as drops. In order to avoid several injections, three vaccines: diphtheria, whooping cough and tetanus (DPT) are combined as single injection. Measles vaccine should be given as soon as after 9 months of age (but not to be given before). The child is usually taken to immunization centre when he/she is one and half months old and after then, every month for DPT and oral polio vaccine. The interval between two doses should not be less than one month. The booster dose of these can be given any time between 16 to 24 months of age. The BCG injection is given within one year. However, while delivery is at hospital BCG and a dose of OPV are given at birth. Tetanus vaccination to pregnant woman protects both child and mother.

As the vaccines require specialized storage conditions for retaining potency, they are carried through cold chain systems and immunization is carried out in a particular day(s) in different centers. Vaccination facilities are available at Anganwadi Centres, Health Sub Centres,

Primary Health Centres, Community Health Centres, District Hospitals and other major hospitals. There are other vaccines too like hepatitis B, MMR etc., but are not covered under universal immunization scheme. However, in some states pentavalent vaccines are included under immunization programme. The pentavalent vaccine is the combination of five vaccines in one: DPT + Hepatitis B + Influenza type B.

National Immunization Schedule (NIS) for Infants, Children and Pregnant Women

Vaccine	When to give	Dose	Route	Site
		For Pregnant Women		
TT-1	Early in pregnancy	0.5 ml	Intra-muscular	Upper Arm
TT-2	4 weeks after TT-1*	0.5 ml	Intra-muscular	Upper Arm
TT- Booster	If received 2 TT doses in a pregnancy within the last 3 yrs*	0.5 ml	Intra-muscular	Upper Arm
		For Infants		
BCG	At birth or as early as possible till one year of age	0.1ml (0.05ml until 1 month age)	Intra-dermal	Left Upper Arm
Hepatitis B - Birth dose	At birth or as early as possible within 24 hours	0.5 ml	Intra-muscular	Antero-lateral side of mid-thigh
OPV-0	At birth or as early as possible within the first 15 days	2 drops	Oral	Oral
OPV 1, 2 & 3	At 6 weeks, 10 weeks & 14 weeks (OPV can be given till 5 years of age)	2 drops	Oral	Oral
Pentavalent 1, 2 & 3	At 6 weeks, 10 weeks & 14 weeks (can be given till one year of age)	0.5 ml	Intra-muscular	Antero-lateral side of mid-thigh
Rotavirus#	At 6 weeks, 10 weeks & 14 weeks (can be given till one year of age)	5 drops	Oral	Oral

Contd...

Vaccine	When to give	Dose	Route	Site
IPV	Two fractional dose at 6 and 14 weeks of age	0.1 ml	Intra dermal two fractional dose	Intra-dermal: Right upper arm
Measles /MR 1st Dose$	9 completed months-12 months. (can be given till 5 years of age)	0.5 ml	Sub-cutaneous	Right upper Arm
JE - 1**	9 completed months-12 months.	0.5 ml	Sub-cutaneous	Left upper Arm
Vitamin A (1st dose)	At 9 completed months with measles-Rubella	1 ml (1 lakh IU)	Oral	Oral
For Children				
DPT booster-1	16-24 months	0.5 ml	Intra-muscular	Antero-lateral side of mid-thigh
Measles/ MR 2nd dose $	16-24 months	0.5 ml	Sub-cutaneous	Right upper Arm
OPV Booster	16-24 months	2 drops	Oral	Oral
JE-2	16-24 months	0.5 ml	Sub-cutaneous	Left Upper Arm
Vitamin A* (2nd to 9th dose)**	16-18 months. Then one dose every 6 months up to the age of 5 years.	2 ml (2 lakh IU)	Oral	Oral
DPT Booster-2	5-6 years	0.5 ml.	Intra-muscular	Upper Arm
TT	10 years & 16 years	0.5 ml	Intra-muscular	Upper Arm

- *Give TT-2 or Booster doses before 36 weeks of pregnancy. However, give these even if more than 36 weeks have passed. Give TT to a woman in labour, if she has not previously received TT.
- **JE Vaccine is introduced in select endemic districts after the campaign.
- *** The 2nd to 9th doses of Vitamin A can be administered to children 1-5 years old during biannual rounds, in collaboration with ICDS.
- #Phased introduction, at present in Andhra Pradesh, Haryana, Himachal Pradesh and Orissa from 2016 & expanded in Madhya Pradesh, Assam, Rajasthan, and Tripura in February 2017 and planned in Tamil Nadu & Uttar Pradesh in 2017.
- $ Phased introduction, at present in five states namely Karnataka, Tamil Nadu, Goa, Lakshadweep and Puducherry. (As of Feb' 2017)

- Vitamin A may also be administered during immunization.

Here are few Practical Tips:

- Vaccinate your child/children on time and be sure that they get complete set of each vaccine they need. Keep the immunization card safely and handy.
- Educate the community too on the benefits of immunization.
- Minor cough, cold or minor fever or diarrhoea are not contraindications for vaccination.
- Do not give DPT to a child with recurrent convulsion or an active neurological disease of central nervous system.
- Do not give DPT –2 and DPT – 3 doses to a child who has had convulsion within three days of most recent dose.
- Do not give BCG to a child with symptomatic HIV infection. But give other vaccines.
- Give all vaccines including BCG to a child with asymptomatic HIV infection.
- Give oral polio drops even if the child has diarrhoea. But the fact should be told to health worker who would arrange for an extra dose later. The dose given during diarrhoea is not counted.

Remember the age-old proverb "Prevention Is Better than Cure". We can prevent the killer diseases through vaccination and make a better and healthier world for our children.

(b) Protect against Seasonal Human Influenza: Get Vaccinated

The seasonal human influenza is a contagious respiratory disease caused by influenza viruses. It can cause mild to severe illness and at times can lead to deaths. As the winter is setting, many people are likely to get affected by this seasonal influenza commonly known as flu.

Influenza affects all age groups. The common symptoms are fever, headache, extreme tiredness, dry cough, sore throat, runny or stuffy nose, muscle aches and stomach symptoms such as nausea, vomiting, diarrhoea. The stomach symptoms are more common in children than adults. Though flu is not life threatening in healthy adults, it can lead to serious complications including deaths in high risk patients. The serious complications include pneumonia, sinus infections, dehydrations and worsening of chronic medical conditions like congestive heart failure, asthma or diabetes. People often confused between common cold and influenza. While cold generally causes a streaming or blocked nose, mild sore throat, headache, or rarely mild fever, the flu is much more severe and cause incapacitating. Flu is very uncomfortable and inconvenient; and is the major cause of absenteeism in office, school or workplace during winter.

Flu viruses spread mainly from person to person through coughing or sneezing of people with influenza. Spread can occur when one touches the objects with flu virus on it and then touches his/her mouth or nose. One can infect others beginning one day before symptoms develop and up to five days after becoming sick. The antiviral drugs are available to treat and prevent flu. They are the second line of defence. The antibiotics do not work against influenza and they are of no value unless bacterial infection occurs at the same time. Vaccination is the best way to prevent influenza.

Vaccination protects.

Influenza vaccine available in our country is flu shot. The flu shot is a killed vaccine and thus one will not get flu from the use of vaccine. The maximum immunity develops after two to three weeks of flu shot (injection). One can get flu even after the flu immunization as it protects only against three types of influenza viruses that could cause serious complications. Flu with other viruses will be milder. The protection lasts for about 9 months. It is necessary to get vaccination every year before beginning of flu season. Though flu vaccination is recommended for all persons above 6 months, these group of persons are at high risk who have a greater need for protection from flu: individuals above 65 years, adults and children with heart diseases, asthma and chronic bronchitis, those under steroid and anticancer medication (as these suppress immune system), persons with diabetes, HIV etc.

Here are the general guidelines for prevention and managing flu (This is different from bird flu):

Prevention

- Consult your doctor to get vaccinated especially you are in the risk group.
- Remember the vaccination may cause some side effects which are usually normal and they will disappear within one to two days. If continues, consult back your doctor.
- Stay at vaccination place for at least 30 minutes after the shot. This is just to check that no untoward reaction occurs.
- Do not take the shot if you have had reactions previously to this vaccine or you have allergy to eggs or egg proteins.
- Do not take if you have fever or a severe infection.
- Avoid close contact with people who are sick.
- Clean your hands frequently and avoid touching your eyes, nose or mouth.

Management (if you have flu)

- Stay at home and take rest.
- Drink plenty of liquids. But avoid alcohol.
- Avoid smoking.
- Take medications to relieve symptoms of flu –
    - Paracetamol or Aspirin to relive fever, headache, and body ache.
    - Do not use aspirin in children without doctor's advice.

  - Steam inhalation is suggested to relieve nasal congestion and tight chest.
  - Gargle with saline water to relieve painful throat.
  - Carefully select your cough syrup for treating cough as there are two types of cough: productive and dry.
- Cover your mouth and nose while coughing and sneezing.
- Do not spread flu by shaking hands or kissing others. The Indian tradition of Namaste (folding hands) is preferable.

CHAPTER 65

Vitamins

(a) Vitamins: How much do We Need?

Vitamins are necessary for good health. They are essential micronutrients required by the body in small quantities. The people with restrictive diets may not get enough of a particular vitamin requiring supplementation. On the other hand, consuming large amounts of vitamins may have harmful effects besides wasting money unnecessarily.

Basically the vitamins are of two types: fat soluble and water soluble. Vitamins A, D, E and K come under fat soluble category and all others: B – Vitamins and vitamin C fall on the later type. B vitamins have several components: thiamine (B_1), riboflavin (B_2), pyridoxine (B_6), cyanocobalamin (B_{12}), niacin, pantothenic acid, biotin (vitamin H) and folic acid. The body can not synthesise most of the vitamins in quantities required for metabolism. They must be supplied by food or supplementation. Vitamin D is an exception.

Vitamin A and E are stored in the body to any extent but vitamin D and K are stored in tiny amounts. Vitamin C is stored in smallest amount and vitamin B_{12} in large amounts. On vitamin supplementation, body either accumulates them or removes them if cannot be stored. While accumulation of more than the required quantities of vitamins may lead to toxic effects, the removal process burdens the liver and kidneys.

The usual daily requirements of various vitamins for an average adult: Vitamin A – 600 microgram (retinal), Vitamin D – 2.5 microgram, Vitamin B_1 – 1.2 mg, Vitamin B_2 – 1.4 mg, Niacin – 16 mg, Vitamin B_6 – 2 mg, Pantothenic acid – 10 mg, Folic acid – 100 microgram, Vitamin B_{12} – 1 microgram and Vitamin C – 60 mg.

Vitamins are useful only if you do have deficiency. Unnecessary use may cause toxicity.

The false hope or superior health or freedom from disease may attract people's attention for taking vitamins. It is often claimed that the present farming methods, poor cooking practice, falling prey to junk foods deprive our bodies of important nutrition including vitamins. Everyone would benefit from vitamin supplementation is a myth. Regular vitamin supplementation is unnecessary unless one has the need. Starvation, disease conditions, eating disorders, alcoholism etc. are primary cause of malnutrition, which may lead to vitamin deficiency. Pregnant or lactating women; growing children; patients undergoing major surgeries, suffering from cancer, severe injury, infection, or trauma are vulnerable and they may be of need.

Each vitamin has a specific function to perform and deficiency of any particular vitamin may lead deficiency disease in our body. No deficiency disease is yet known for vitamin E. Vitamin A deficiency is considered a public health problem in our country. Its deficiency increases the severity and the risks of three main health threats facing children: diarrhoeal diseases, measles and pneumonia. The deficiency causes ophthalmic problems too (night blindness). On the other hand, large amount of vitamin A can cause loss of appetite, itching, skin disorders, loss of weight, enlargement of liver and spleen etc.

Vitamin D is derived both from sunlight and food. Its deficiency leads to rickets (bone disorder), a condition usually observed in young children. Excessive dose of vitamin D can cause serious problems. It produces rise in blood calcium, which can cause debility, drowsiness, nausea, abdominal pain, thirst, constipation, nausea, deposits of calcium in various tissues and organs, kidney damage and kidney stones.

The deficiency of vitamin E is extremely rare. It is primarily an antioxidant in protecting cellular membranes from oxidative damage or destruction. It is relatively non-toxic. Vitamin K deficiency can cause bleeding disorder and is used only under medical supervision. It is partly supplied by dietary intake and microbial synthesis in the gut.

Vitamin B_1 deficiency may result in beri-beri. Vitamin B_2 deficiency may occur in association with other vitamin B complex deficiency states (pellagra). Vitamin B_6 deficiency is rare as the vitamin is widely distributed in foods, but deficiency may occur during isonizid therapy (Tuberculosis). Nicotinic acid inhibits the synthesis of cholesterol and used in deficiency (pellagra). The deficiency of folic acid is associated with megaloblastic anaemia. Supplementation to women of child bearing potential is recommended. Vitamin C is used to prevent and treat scurvy. The value of vitamin C in the treatment of common colds is unsubstantiated.

The water soluble vitamins readily pass out of the body when excessive amounts are taken, so adverse effects are minimised. Doses of vitamin C greater than 1 gram a day may cause diarrhoea. It often disturbs the result of common blood tests. The interference of vitamin C with the functioning of some contraceptives is also reported. Vitamin B_6 in large doses has been reported to cause serious nerve damage.

The pharmaceutical market is flooded with many vitamin preparations and often as multivitamin products. Many of these are irrational and undesirable too. This poses unnecessary threat to our health and additional financial burden to our pockets. Do not get misled by advertisement. Vitamins may be required to supplement an inadequate diet but never to complement a diet.

Remember the hard facts:

- Vitamin supplements are not the substitutes of good nutrition.
- Vitamin preparations are medicine too. Keep them away from children.
- Do not self medicate unless you are sure of their supplementation. Consult your doctor or neighbourhood pharmacist.
- Take them with meals if experience gastro intestinal effects.
- Some of the vitamins influence the effect of other medicines. Tell your doctor that you are taking these products.
- Unnecessary use of vitamins not only can cause toxic effects, they too empty your pocket. Body can utilize them only if there is requirement or deficiency.

(b) Vitamin A

Measles is one of the major causes of childhood morbidity and mortality. Vitamin A deficiency is a risk factor for severe measles infection. Measles is caused by a virus and results in high fever and risk. Possible complications include pneumonia. World Health Organization recommends the administration of an oral dose of vitamin A 200,000 International Units (IU) each day for two days in children with measles when they live in areas where vitamin A deficiency may be present.

Vitamin A is a group of fat soluble compounds essential for vision, growth, reproduction, cellular differentiation and proliferation and integrity of the immune system. It is known by different names like: β carotene, retinoic acid. Most of the body's vitamin is in the liver. Vitamin A deficiency is rare in well nourished population and develops slowly because of body's store. It is most common in poorly nourished children below 5 years of age. The first symptom of vitamin A deficiency is usually night blindness. If left untreated, a foamy deposit may appear in the white of the eye and the cornea may harden causing xerophthalmia, a condition can lead to permanent blindness.

Other deficiency disorders include increased susceptibility to infection, follicular keratosis, loss of appetite, impaired taste and smell. Vitamin A deficiency also produces inflammation of the skin (cracked skin).

The normal daily requirement of vitamin A

Categories	Amount per day
Children 4-6 years	2500 IU
Adult male	5000 IU
Adult female	4000 IU
Pregnant women	5000 IU
Lactating mothers	6000 IU

Do not exceed recommended dose. Excess intake may cause accumulation in the body.

Vitamin requirements increases above normal in the below mentioned situation: cystic fibrosis, chronic diarrhoea, obstruction of bile duct, over active thyroid gland and long use of lipid lowering medicines. Pregnant and breast feeding women need extra vitamin A for themselves and their babies. Children with measles are at high risk of xerophthalmia. Vitamin A should be given moment illness begins. Giving vitamin A supplements to HIV infected women might make it likely that their children would be infected with HIV. Mother to child transmission of HIV is the primary way that children become infected with HIV. Vitamin A analogues are reported to have value in preventing and treating certain cancers and treating certain skin disorders.

Vitamin A is available in plenty in food source. Dark green leafy vegetables, yellow or red fruits and vegetables, whole milk, eggs, liver and kidneys are rich in vitamin A. One large carrot contains around 11,000 IU of vitamin A.

Vitamin A is available as sugar coated tablets, capsules, syrups and injections. The dose for suggested for prevention and treatment of deficiency:

Purpose	Categories of patients	Dose
Prevention	Infant, under 6 months	50 000 units
	Infant, 6-12 months	100 000 units every 4-6 months, preferably at measles vaccination.
	Child over 1 year	200 000 units every 4-6 months
	Adult	200 000 units every 6 months
	Adult Pregnant women	Maximum 10 000 units daily or maximum 25 000 units weekly.
	Adult mothers	200 000 units at delivery or within 6 weeks.
Treatment of xerophthalmia	Infant under 6 months	50 000 units on diagnosis, repeated next day and then after 2 weeks
	Infant, 6-12 months	100 000 immediately on diagnosis, repeated next day and then after 2 weeks.
	Child over 1 year and adult (except women of child bearing age)	200 000 units on diagnosis, repeated next day and then after 2 weeks.
	Women of child bearing age (adult)	Consult your doctor as high intake of may cause birth defects.

Unlike water soluble vitamins, Vitamin A is not eliminated from the body. The excess than the body's requirements get accumulated often to dangerous and toxic levels in the body. The toxic effects of excessive vitamin A include liver damage, weakness, increased pressure in the brain, bone and joint pain, damage, dry and rough skin. Some of the chronic toxicity problems of vitamin A are reversible on cessation of intake. β carotene found in carrot is converted slowly into vitamin A in the body and can be consumed without causing toxicity. The diagnosis of vitamin A toxicity is based on symptoms and on abnormal high level of vitamin A in the blood.

Few general guidelines:

- Deficiency, if identified or diagnosed properly, can be treated with Vitamin A preparations. If problem persists or continues, consult your doctor.
- As it is associated with birth defects, it should be given in smaller doses (no more than 10000 units per day) to women of child bearing age. Do not self medicate. Consult your doctor.
- Use oral preparations as first preference. They are cheap and much safer than injections. The injections are costly and painful.
- Like all other medicines, keep them out of reach of children.

(c) Vitamin B Complex

Vitamin B composed various water soluble vitamins collectively called Vitamin B Complex. This includes at least Thiamine (Vitamin B_1), Riboflavin (Vitamin B_2), Pyridoxine (Vitamin B_6) and Nicotinamide. They are also available as single product.

Vitamin B_1 is essential in a number of physiological processes involving enzymes including release of energy from glucose. The important sources of this vitamin are whole grain cereals, wheat, gram, yeast, pulses, oilseeds and groundnut. Smaller amounts are also available in meat, fish, eggs, vegetables and fruits. The polished rice has no thiamine and is lost during milling. Boiled rice (parboiling) is better than raw rice. Boiling the rice before husking disperses the vitamin throughout the grain.

The deficiency of thiamine can occur due to inadequate vitamin in the diet, chronic diarrhoea (reduces absorption), hyperthyroidism (requirement of increased need), pregnancy and severe alcoholism. The early deficiency symptoms include fatigue, irritability, memory impairment, loss of appetite, sleep disturbances, abdominal discomfort and weight loss. The two principal deficiency diseases are beriberi and Wernicke-Korsakoff syndrome. Beriberi begins as a prickling sensation in the toes, a burning sensation in the feet becoming severe at night, muscle cramps in the calves, and pain in legs and feet. The affect on heart are high output of blood from heart, a fast heart rate, and dilation of blood vessels, causing the skin to be warm and moist. Wernicke-Korsakoff's encephalopathy, also known as cerebral beriberi, has the symptoms like mental confusion, laryngitis, and double vision etc.

The recommended dose is 10-25 mg daily by mouth for mild chronic thiamine deficiency. Injections are available for severe deficiency states. The allergic reactions may occur on injections which include skin inflammation and other hypersensitive reactions including anaphylaxis. The injection may cause tenderness and tissue changes at injection site. In severe cases, it may even cause respiratory distress, gastrointestinal bleeding, vascular collapse and death.

Vitamin B_2 (Riboflavin) is involved in cellular oxidation. It is important in many cell processes leading to energy production and amino acid metabolism. The richest dietary sources are milk, eggs, liver, kidney and greeny leafy vegetables. Germination increases the riboflavin content of pulses and cereals. Polished rice is deficient of this vitamin.

The riboflavin deficiency may occur from reduced dietary intake or reduced absorption due to liver disease, alcoholism, chronic infection or probenecid therapy (often used with penicillin therapy). It may also occur in association with other deficiency states like pellagra (Deficiency associated with Nicotinamide). The most common symptoms of deficiency are sores in the corner of the mouth, cracks on the lips. If thrush, a yeast infection may develop in these areas and grayish-white patches may occur. The tongue may turn magenta (purplish red) and greasy.

The usual of dose of riboflavin is up to 30 mg in divided dose (by mouth) for the treatment of vitamin B_2 deficiency. The prophylaxis dose is 1-2 mg daily. Large amount of riboflavin taken orally may cause diarrhoea and frequent urination with yellow orange discolouration of urine.

Vitamin B_3 (Niacin/Nicotinamide): Niacin is essential for the metabolism of carbohydrates, fat and proteins; for the normal functioning of the skin, intestinal and nervous system. This inhibits the synthesis of cholesterol and triglyceride and is useful in the treatment of some hyperlipidaemias. Nicotinic acid and Nicotinamide are used to prevent and treat nicotinic acid deficiency.

The rich sources of this vitamin are liver, kidney meat, poultry, fish, legumes, and ground nut. The deficiency causes pellagra and is characterized by diarrhoea, dermatitis and dementia. Glossitis and stomatitis may also occur.

The usual dose of niacin for treating pellagra is up to 500 mg daily in divided dose. It is not to be used in patients with liver dysfunction, active peptic ulcer, severe hypotension, arterial haemorrhage or hypersensitivity. The most of the adverse effects are dose dependent. The patients are advised: to take the medicine with meals to minimize gastric irritation; to avoid hot liquids when initially taking to reduce flushing response; and not to make sudden postural changes to minimize effects of orthostatic hypotension.

The B group of vitamins are useful if there are deficiencies. The excess get eliminated easily.

Pyridoxine (Vitamin B_6) deficiency is rare as this is widely distributed in foods but deficiency may occur during isoniazid therapy (Tuberculosis) and is characterized by peripheral neuritis. The good sources of pyridoxine are milk, liver, meat, egg yolk, fish, whole grain cereals, legumes and vegetables. High doses are advised in some metabolic disorders such as hyperoxaluria and in sideroblastic anaemia. Pyridoxine and thiamine are also useful in status epilepticus. It is also useful for treating nausea and vomiting during pregnancy.

The dose of pyridoxine: 25-50 mg up to 3 times daily (oral) for treatment of deficiency; 10 mg daily (prophylaxis) and 50 mg 3 times daily (treatment) in isoniazid neuropathy; 100 to 400 mg daily in divided doses in sideroblastic anaemia. Pyridoxine is generally well tolerated but chronic administration of high doses may cause peripheral neuritis.

These are the general guidelines:

- Do not believe the advertisements which claim that many of your health problems can be solved by vitamin supplements.
- Vitamin supplementation is not the substitute of good and nutritious food. Eating good food is the best way to improve nutritional health.
- Though B vitamins normally pass out of the body in urine, the high doses may cause adverse effects. Vitamin B_6 is associated with nerve damage.
- Do not take mega doses without doctor's advice.

(d) B – Complex Vitamins: Diet a Better Source

The vitamins neither supply energy nor do they contribute to the building of tissues; but are extremely essential for a variety of body responses including energy production, use of mineral and growth of healthy tissues. While the oil soluble vitamins (Vitamin A, D, E and K) get accumulated in the body when intake is more than the required, the water soluble vitamins (Vitamin B – Complex and Vitamin C) get easily eliminated from the body when taken more than the required. Thus water soluble vitamins are safer but not free from toxicities. The B-Complex Vitamins consists of eight water soluble vitamins. They are: thiamin, riboflavin, niacin, pantothenic acid, pyridoxine, folate, cyanocobalamin, and biotin.

Thiamin (also known as vitamin B_1): Thiamin is one of the most important B-Complex vitamins and is useful for initiating many metabolic reactions. It is essential for the health of nerve tissues and for normal cardiac and gastrointestinal functions. Since it plays an important role in carbohydrate metabolism, its dietary need depends on energy intake. Deficiency occurs around 3 weeks after intake of thiamin is stopped. Severe neurological problems arise in chronic and severe alcoholics due to thiamin deficiency as often they go without food for long time. Highly processed food stuff like white bread, polished rice, refined sugar are deficient in thiamin.

Inadequate diet, alcoholism, malabsorption syndrome, prolonged diarrhoea, pregnancy and food faddism may cause deficiency of thiamin which may require supplementation.

Riboflavin (also known as vitamin B_2): This yellow looking vitamin involves in numerous oxidation-reduction process in the body. The cellular growth cannot occur without this vitamin. It promotes normal growth; assists in the synthesis of steroids, RBC, and glycogen; helps in maintenance of mucous membrane, eyes, nervous system; and aids in iron absorption. We get yellow coloured urine after taking vitamin B complex is because of this riboflavin.

Cereals and pulses are poor sources of riboflavin. But the germination increases their riboflavin content. Its deficiency occurs along with deficiency of other B group of vitamins.

Niacin (also known as vitamin B_3 or Nicotinic acid): It accepts or donates hydrogen in the aerobic respiration of all body cells. This is a different vitamin which body synthesizes from dietary tryptophan. It also helps in lowering triglycerides and low density lipoproteins. The high lipid level is a risk factor for heart diseases. It does not get excreted as it is but only after metabolism.

Pantothenic acid (also known as vitamin B_5): Pantothenic acid helps in cholesterol, steroid and fatty acid synthesis. It is widely distributed in plants and animal tissues and hence its deficiency is rare and difficult to diagnose.

Pyridoxine (also known as vitamin B_6): Pyridoxine is the most important form of Vitamin B_6 of three forms. It plays an important role in the metabolism of amino acids, fats and carbohydrates. The deficiency occurs from poor absorption from gastrointestinal tract or the use of medicines like isoniazid (TB medicine) that deplete vitamin B_6. The excessive dose can severely damage nerves, destroying part of the spinal cord which makes the walking difficult.

Folic acid: Folic acid and B_{12} vitamin work interdependently in the formation of normal red blood cells and in the production of an essential building block of DNA. The deficiency causes anemia. Folic acid deficiency usually occurs during pregnancy especially when diets are lack of green leafy vegetables and legumes. The pregnant women are given iron and folic acid tablets free to prevent deficiency related issues.

Cyanocobalamin (also known as vitamin B_{12}): This is the most complex vitamin molecule and is available in the body as methylcobalamin, hydroxycobalamin, and adenosylcobalamin. It is active in all cells especially those in the bone marrow, central nervous system, and gastrointestinal tract. It helps in methylation reaction and cell division in association with folic acid. As it is involved in metabolism of folates, folate deficiency appears as a feature of B_{12} deficiency. Vitamin B_{12} is produced exclusively by microorganisms and available in animal protein. Very little is available in some vegetables due to the presence of microbes. The vegetarians who consume no animal products are at risk of developing B_{12} deficiency.

Biotin (also known as vitamin H): It plays active role in fat, amino acid and carbohydrate metabolism. In addition to dietary sources, colonic flora contributes to the amount of biotin in the body. Those who take raw egg whites are at risk of deficiency. White of raw egg contains a protein (avidin) that binds biotin and prevents absorption.

Vitamin	Deficiency causes	Dietary / Natural Sources	Toxicity of excess intake
Vitamin B_1	Beriberi [muscle wasting, mental confusion, anorexia, enlarged heart, nerve changes]	Whole grain, coarse brown rice, pork, beef, fresh peas and beans.	Rapid pulse, weakness, headache, insomnia, irritability
Vitamin B_2	Cracks at corners of mouth, sore throat, skin rash, hypersensitivity to light, purple tongue	Meat, poultry, fish, dairy products, green vegetables.	Not known but interferes with anti-cancer medication.
Vitamin B_3	Pellagra [diarrhoea, irritability, loss of appetite, weakness, mental confusion progressing to psychosis, dermatitis.]	Lean meats, fish, liver, cereals, whole grains, green vegetables.	Diarrhoea, nausea, vomiting, flushing of the skin, liver dysfunction and glucose intolerance
Vitamin B_5 [Pantothenic acid]	Vomiting, intestinal distress, insomnia, fatigue, numbness and tingling of hands and feet.	Liver, yeast, vegetables	Occasional diarrhoea, water retention
Vitamin B_6	Anemia, cracked corner of the mouth, irritability, muscle twitching, dermatitis, nausea, confusion, kidney stone	Meat, cereals, lentils, nuts, potatoes, bananas.	Bloating, headache, fatigue, depression, damage to nerves leading to loss of reflexes and sensation, walking difficulty
Folic acid	Anaemia, weakness, fatigue, irritability, shortness of breath, swollen tongue	Green leafy vegetables, pulses, cereals, liver, kidney, mushroom, yeast.	Diarrhoea, insomnia, irritability, masking of Vit B_6 deficiency symptoms, may increase the frequency of seizure in epileptic patients.

Contd....

Vitamin	Deficiency causes	Dietary / Natural Sources	Toxicity of excess intake
Vitamin B_{12}	Anaemia, fatigue, degeneration of peripheral nerves progressing to paralysis, hypersensitivity of the skin	Meat, fish, egg and milk products. [Not available in vegetable food]	Not known
Biotin	Abnormal heart action, loss of appetite, nausea, depression, muscle pain, weakness, fatigue, drying, scary dermatitis, hair loss	Liver, kidneys, egg yolk, yeast, cauliflower, nuts, legumes.	Not known

As B-Complex vitamins are water soluble, they quickly dissolve in water. One needs to be careful not to lose them during cooking or processing. Over cooking causes loss of these vitamins from the diet. Longer the fresh vegetables are steamed or boiled; much would be the loss of vitamins. In order to have adequate amounts of vitamins, it is necessary to eat a variety of food. With balanced diets, enough vitamins are obtained for a healthy living. The extra supplementation through food supplements and vitamin tablets or tonics is not only unnecessary but also be expensive. However some conditions may require supplementation: deficiency condition, pregnancy, lactation, infancy or elderly. It is preferable to discuss with the doctors before starting these vitamins for daily use.

(e) Fight Diseases with Vitamin C

Bleeding under the skin particularly around hair follicles, under finger nails, around the gums and into the joints are some of the deficiency symptoms of vitamin C. the person may become depressed, tired and weak. Bleeding, loose teeth, inflammation of gums are known as scurvy, deficiency disease of vitamin C.

Vitamin C is also known as ascorbic acid and is essential for the formation of connective tissues that hold the body's structure together. It helps binds cells together and promotes healing. It also assists in the absorption of non-heme iron from food by reducing the ferric iron. But it is the most easily destroyed of all vitamins.

Vitamin C has been called as 'fresh food' vitamin. The rich dietary source for it includes citrus fruits, tomatoes, potatoes, cabbage and green peppers. Meat, fish, poultry, eggs too contain some vitamin C, but is generally absent in grains. A medium sized orange contains around 60 mg vitamin C. The recommended daily allowance for adult is around 60 mg per day.

The dose of vitamin as recommended:

Prophylaxis of scurvy, by mouth, adult and child 25-75 mg daily; Treatment of scurvy, by mouth, adult and child not less than 250 mg daily in divided doses.

Vitamin C has versatile activity.

Ascorbic acid has been reported to have beneficial effects in common cold: to prevent or lessen the severity of cold. The high doses of vitamin C has been suggested as remedies for many conditions: from common cold to cancer. But there is little evidence that taking vitamin C prevents diseases. However, vitamin C supplementation may have preventive effects in populations with high incidence of pneumonia and may have therapeutic benefits in populations with low plasma vitamin C levels.

Higher doses of vitamin may cause the following side effects: diarrhoea, flushing or redness of the skin, headache, and mild increase in urination, nausea or vomiting, stomach cramps. Excessive use of chewable tablets has reported to cause breakdown of tooth enamel. High doses of vitamin C may also be harmful in certain circumstances. Ascorbic acid toxicity may increase oxalate excretion causing chances of kidney stones. The high dose is also risky for people who use anticoagulants. It may also cause changes in menstrual cycle. Rebound scurvy may develop if suddenly stopped high doses.

Here are the general guidelines for safe and effective use of vitamin C:

- While self medication with vitamin C never take more than the recommended daily allowance. High doses products are not only expensive; they have limited beneficial effects except in scurvy.
- While taking high doses, reduce your dose gradually. Body needs to adjust.
- If you miss a dose, take as soon as you remember, but skip it if it is almost time for next dose. Do not take double doses.
- Tell your doctor that you are taking vitamin C. It interferes with glucose test. High doses even may interfere with test for blood in your stool.
- Consult your doctor or health care professional, before taking vitamin C if you have kidney stone problem.
- Like all other medicines, keep them away from children.

(f) Vitamin C – a Vitamin for Many Conditions!

Vitamin C (also known as ascorbic acid) is the most unstable vitamin and is not produced in human body. This needs to be taken from outside. Other animals excluding monkeys and guinea pigs synthesize this vitamin and they do not have deficiency. Only humans, monkeys and guinea pigs do need to ingest the vitamin failing which they develop a condition called scurvy. It is present in all body tissues but at a higher concentration in adrenal glands, pituitary gland, and intestinal wall. Vitamin C has been promoted to have beneficial effects in wide range of conditions from common cold to tuberculosis to cancer. Some of these effects are not significant enough to support the use of vitamin C as therapy. It is required for the formation of collagen (main structural protein of mammalian connective tissue) and thus useful for the formation and maintenance of connective tissues, bones, tendons, skin, teeth and capillaries. It is a good antioxidant and thus useful in free radical scavenging.

The vitamin C is called fresh food vitamin. It is widely available in nature and the rich sources are: fruits like amlas, lemons, oranges, guavas, pineapples, mangoes, banana; and green leafy vegetables and tomatoes. Milk and meat contains very little. It is absent in grains. The vitamin C is rapidly oxidized in presence of air and destroyed by heat. It is for this reason; much of the vitamin is lost from the vegetables when they are dry, stale or cut and exposed to air. The vitamin C content of fruits and vegetables is reduced by storage and damage to plant cells by rough handling, bruising or cutting. Even the deep fried potatoes have more vitamin C compared to boiled ones due to air exposure. Human milk contains 3 to 4 times as much vitamin C as that of cow's milk. Heat and pasteurization further reduce the vitamin C content in cow's milk. The fermentation cooking process such as making idli, dosa and dhokla have increased nutrients with vitamin B complex and vitamin C.

Vitamin C deficiency is rare and the deficiency causes a condition called scurvy [see box]. Scurvy can be easily prevented and treated by increasing the intake of vitamin C in diet or using a supplement. The supplement is necessary only when the diet does not contain enough vitamin C, or when one requires more vitamin C due to surgery, smoking or infectious diseases. The women taking contraceptives may require extra vitamin C. The recommended dietary intake of ascorbic acid is 40 g per day for adults, children (excluding infants), 60 mg per day for pregnant women and 80 mg per day lactating mothers. High intake through supplementation does not help except in persons with scurvy. High doses are not only expensive; they may cause serious health risk. It may increase oxalate excretion (risk in patients with kidney stone) and lead to haemolysis in patients deficient in glucose – 6-phosphate dehydrogenase (a hereditary disease).

The supplementation of vitamin C may improve the general health and well being. But one should avoid self medicating with mega doses. As ascorbic acid promotes the absorption of dietary iron, the regular intake of the vitamin is suggested. The citrus fruits are good source for our daily requirements of vitamin C.

Scurvy had been a cause of suffering for thousands of years. It killed more sailors than the battles, storms and other diseases combined from the 16th to 18th centuries. It was Dr. James Lind's experiment on 12 sailors that found orange and lemons as the remedy of scurvy. Scurvy is a condition characterised by swollen and bleeding gums, loosen teeth, muscle and joint pain, failure of wounds to heal, anaemia and weakness. James Lind was a Scottish doctor and was an expert in naval hygiene. In 1747, while serving as surgeon he identified 12 sailors with serious scurvy and divided them into six groups. Each group was given the same food but supplemented with different substances thought to be the remedies. One group was given oranges and lemon and this group showed a remarkable recovery. This experiment led to the discovery of lemons and oranges as remedy of scurvy. The experiment of James Lind is regarded as one of the earliest scientific experiments in medical sciences. Though Lind's experiment and publications proved the usefulness of citrus fruits in managing scurvy, it took almost another 40 years to practice and provide these fruits as a part of diet in navy.

Scurvy is no longer an important health issue like earlier as the source of vitamin C is widely available in nature.

CHAPTER 66

Anti-Emetic Medicines (Medicines for Vomiting)

Vomiting is a sign of many different problems. This may result from the problems in the stomach or gut such as infection, food poisoning, appendicitis. Vomiting may also occur in malaria, hepatitis, tonsillitis, earache, meningitis, urinary infection, gall bladder pain or migraine headache.

Nausea and vomiting are caused by the activation of the vomiting centre in the brain. Nausea refers the unpleasant feeling in the abdomen that often ends with vomiting while vomiting refers to forceful expulsion of stomach contents through the mouth. Vomiting is one of the methods the body uses to eliminate the harmful substances. Though the person feels unwell while vomiting, generally it provides some comfort after vomiting. The anti-emetic medicines help preventing or treating vomiting symptoms. But it is necessary to find the causes of the vomiting and address them. One should look at the following danger signs which may warrant immediate medical attention: increased dehydration; severe vomiting; vomits of dark green, brown or smells like shit; constant pain in the gut; blood vomiting.

In general, mild vomiting may be treated with oral medicines but severe vomiting requires injections.

Promethazine

It is available as tablet, syrup and injection. It is useful in treating motion sickness and nausea. It has limited effect on chemotherapy mild to moderate vomiting. Being antihistamine, it is also useful in the treatment of rhinitis (running nose) and to cause sedation. The common side effects of this medicine are sedation, confusion, sleepiness, dizziness, disorientation, extra-pyramidal symptoms, drowsiness, blurred vision, nausea and vomiting, dry mouth etc.

While taking promethazine do not involve in activities requiring high alertness as driving.

This should be used with caution in patients with asthma, cardiac, pulmonary or hepatic disease. The general guidelines for its safe and effective use are:

- The usual adult dose: motion sickness – 25 mg twice daily; and for nausea – 12.5 to 25 mg orally repeated at intervals of not less than 4 hours (with maximum 100 mg in 24 hour). For motion sickness – take at bedtime before travel, repeat on the day of travel as necessary.
- Take with food or meal. If vomiting, swallow with little water and nothing else should be swallowed for 5 minutes.
- Take the first dose 30-60 minutes before travelling.
- Do not take the second dose until the dehydration has been corrected.
- Avoid alcohol during taking this medicine.
- Do not use during breast feeding.
- Do not take when you are using the other medicines like anti-anxiety agents, barbiturates, sleeping tablets or other anti-histamines. There may be additive effects.
- Do not involve yourself in performing skilled tasks like operating heavy machineries or driving. This medicine may impair your ability or alertness.
- Do not expose yourself to Sun as photosensitive reactions may occur.

Metoclopramide

Metoclopramide is available as tablet or injection. It is an anti-vomiting medicine and is useful against nausea and vomiting associated with gastrointestinal disorders or migraine, following surgery and chemotherapy. It is also effective against radiation induced nausea and vomiting. It is not effective in the prevention or treatment of motion sickness.

Avoid high alertness activities like driving.

This medicine is not to be used in patients with gastrointestinal obstruction, haemorrhage, or perforations, immediate post gastrointestinal surgery, and convulsive disorder. It should be used with caution in patients with history of depression, Parkinson's disease and hypertension. The common adverse effects of this medicine are: extra-pyramidal symptoms (inability to initiate movement, inability to remain motionless) in children and young adults, drowsiness, restlessness, dizziness, headache, diarrhoea, depression, hypotension and hypertension. The extra-pyramidal reactions occur shortly after treatment and subside within 24 hours of withdrawal of the medicine.

The general guidelines for safe and effective use of Metoclopramide as anti-emetic medicine:

- The usual adult dose 10 mg three times a day. [High doses are necessary in cancer chemotherapy].
- Take this medicine 30 minutes before each meal.
- The product is light sensitive. Do not expose the product to direct sunlight.
- Avoid alcohol use. This would increase central nervous system depression.
- Do not drive at least for 2 hours after dosing.
- Report the side effects like twitching or involuntary movement to your doctor as you experience them.

CHAPTER 67

Cosmetics Use

(a) Cosmetics User – Beware!

Someone once said “We make cosmetics in our factory but we sell hopes in the store”. With this hope people continue using them in attempt to improve their appearances. We all get fascinated by the endorsement of many of these products by our celebrity film actors. But the recent startling findings on the presence of toxic heavy metals in the cosmetics raised serious concern on this hope and safety of such products. Centre for Science and Environment, a not for profit organization, recently tested the marketed cosmetics and revealed the presence of mercury in 44 percent of fairness cream, chromium in 50 percent and nickel in 43 percent of lipstick samples tested.

The import and manufacturing of cosmetics are regulated under the Drugs and Cosmetics Act. Though the cosmetics were not under the purview of initial statute ‘Drugs Act 1940’, following the reports of ill effects of harmful cosmetics they were brought under control with the amendment and renaming the original statute as ‘Drugs and Cosmetics Act’ in 1962. However, the standards of cosmetics are not well defined. The Bureau of Indian Standard (BIS) just defines the requirements of colours and limits the extent of arsenic, lead and other heavy metals in the permitted synthetic and natural colours. The present revelation shows that 14 of the 32 tested fairness has the presence of mercury from 0.10 parts per million (ppm) to 1.97 ppm. 15 out of 30 tested lipsticks showed the presenceof 0.45 ppm to 17.83 ppm of chromium and 13 out of 30 lipstick products found to have nickel in the range of 0.57 to 9.18 ppm. The content of heavy metals in these cosmetic products are much higher than the permissible limits.

Mercury in any form is highly toxic and potentially dangerous for pregnant woman, foetus and child. Exposure to mercury, even in fairly small amounts, may cause serious health issues. Mercury may have toxic effects on the nervous, digestive and immune system, and on lungs, kidneys and eyes. Mercury released to environment is eaten by fishes. The individuals eating such fishes expose themselves to mercurial toxicities. Realising the toxicity of mercury based products and their environmental impact, worldwide it has been advocated to discontinue the use of mercury based health products. Even in Delhi, the Government has initiated steps even to replace the mercury based clinical thermometers with digital ones. One can just imagine the health impact of use of such fairness products. The other two heavy metals found in lip sticks are equally hazardous too. Chromium is known to be carcinogenic and the acute ingestion of nickel is known to cause nausea, vomiting, diarrhoea and headache. Nickel too is a known carcinogenic and can cause several harmful effects even deaths. The lipsticks are invariably gets ingested by users.

Though the products of both Indian as well as multinational foreign brands do have heavy metals, there is some good news too. Not that all the cosmetics tested have the toxic heavy metals. 56 percent of the products do not have mercury content. But this raises another concern: when some products are free from heavy toxic metals why do others have. Is it that there is lack of clear cut standard or lack of implementation of regulatory measures for this lapse? The manufacturing companies have taken it granted to our inadequate implementation of regulatory measures. This is not the first time health concern of cosmetics become an issue. In couple of years before, precisely 2009, the around 100 women complained of skin inflammation and pain following the use of mehendi on their palms as a part of Id celebration in several districts of Odisha. The Government needs to enforce the regulation in the interest of public safety on cosmetics use. The Central Consumer Protection Council now proposes for a compensatory provision for false and misleading claims of cosmetics. Even the celebrities endorsing such products would be made liable for such misleading advertisements. Let's wish the cosmetics would bring more hope than the safety concern!

(b) Darker Side of Skin Care Products!

"The recent compensation of USD 72 million granted by an US Court to the family of an Alabama woman (USA) who died from ovarian cancer which was linked to well-known baby powder and other products containing talcum" raises serious concern about the safety aspects of cosmetics. She was reported to have used iconic talcum powder as a bathroom staple for decades which caused the cancer, her cause of death.

Indian market is flooded with many skin care or cosmetic products of doubtful efficacy and do have potential to cause damaging effect to health. Here is a case of fairness cream, a cocktail mixture, for the men who are in pursuit of fair skin. Flucinolone is a steroid used to treat the itching, redness, dryness, crusting, scaling, inflammation, and discomfort of various skin conditions; Hydroquinone is a skin bleaching agent; and Tretinoin is a form of Vitamin A helps skin to renew quickly. This is a steroid based cream and un-necessary and prolong use can cause serious adverse effects. "Facial erythema with skin irritation, aggravation of acne, and steroid addiction" are the main adverse effects reported by many studies. The dermatologists cautioned against the unsupervised use of these creams.

Hydroquinone lightens the areas of darken skin by decreasing the production and increasing the breakdown of melanin in skin. Melanin is responsible for skin pigmentation. It requires at least a month or so to see the effects of topical hydroquinone in lightening the skin. Though topical use of hydroquinone is often well tolerated, some users may experience minor and temporary skin irritations like mild itching and reddening of the skin. Tretinoin is indicated for the treatment of acne. It controls but not cures. It takes about two to three weeks to see a visible change of improvement. However, it may also cause warmth or slight stinging of the skin, scaling of skin, increase in acne sores, blistering or crusting of the skin.

Another startling finding is the presence of heavy metals in fairness creams. The Centre for Science and Environment, a not for profit organization, recently tested the marketed cosmetics and revealed the presence of mercury in 44 % of fairness creams. Other cosmetics are no less hazardous. The presence of chromium in 50 % and nickel in 43 % of lipstick samples are also detected. The present revelation showed that 14 of the 32 tested fairness has the presence of mercury from 0.10 parts per million (ppm) to 1.97 ppm. 15 out of 30 tested lipsticks showed the presence of 0.45 ppm to 17.83 ppm of chromium and 13 out of 30 lipstick products found to have nickel in the range of 0.57 to 9.18 ppm. The content of heavy metals in these cosmetic products are much higher than the permissible limits.

Mercury in any form is highly toxic and potentially dangerous for pregnant woman, foetus and child. Exposure to mercury, even in fairly small amounts, may cause serious health issues. Mercury may have toxic effects on the nervous, digestive and immune system, and on lungs, kidneys and eyes. Mercury released to environment is eaten by fishes. The individuals eating such fishes expose themselves to mercurial toxicities. Realising the toxicity of mercury based products and their environmental impact, worldwide it has been advocated to discontinue the use of mercury based health products. The steps are initiated by various authorities even to replace the mercury based clinical thermometers with digital ones. One can just imagine the health impact of use of such fairness products. The other two heavy metals found in lip sticks are equally hazardous too. Chromium is known to be carcinogenic and the acute ingestion of nickel is known to cause nausea, vomiting, diarrhoea and headache. Nickel too is a known carcinogenic and can cause several harmful effects even deaths. The lipsticks are invariably gets ingested by users. The baby shampoo was also known to contain harmful ingredients.

Someone once said "We make cosmetics in our factory but we sell hopes in the store". The industry should be conscious enough to selling hopes but not harming the users.

(c) Ugly Truths of Your Fairness Creams!

In India (perhaps in many other countries too) we have an obsession with fair skin. With changing trends, men too started showing their attention for beauty products to make themselves more attractive. Advertisement market is flooded with "an ideal cream for you" type advertisements seducing you to use these products. Many of these products are of doubtful efficacy and do have potential to cause damaging effect to your health. Two recent media reports raised a serious concern on the safety of these products.

Recently the entire stock of a cream containing flucinolone, hydroquinone and tretinoin promoted as a fairness cream for men is seized by the Food and Drug Administration of Maharashtra citing violation of two laws of the country: Drugs and Cosmetics Act; and Drug and Magic Remedies (Objectionable Advertisement) Act. The cream is a cocktail mixture for the men who are in pursuit of fair skin. Flucinolone is a steroid used to treat the itching, redness, dryness, crusting, scaling, inflammation, and discomfort of various skin conditions; Hydroquinone is a skin bleaching agent; and Tretinoin is a form of Vitamin Ahelps skin to renew quickly. This is a steroid based cream and un-necessary and prolong use can cause serious adverse effects. "Facial erythema with skin irritation, aggravation of acne, and steroid addiction" are the main adverse effects reported by many studies. The dermatologists argue against the unsupervised use of these creams.

Hydroquinone lightens the areas of darken skin by decreasing the production and increasing the breakdown of melanin in skin. Melanin is responsible for skin pigmentation. It requires at least a month or so to see the effects of topical hydroquinone in lightening the skin. Though topical use of hydroquinone is often well tolerated, some users may experience minor and temporary skin irritations like mild itching and reddening of the skin. Tretinoin is indicated for the treatment of acne. It controls but not cures. It takes about two to three weeks to see a visible change of improvement. However, it may also cause warmth or slight stinging of the skin, scaling of skin, increase in acne sores, blistering or crusting of the skin.

Another startling finding is the presence of heavy metals in fairness creams. The Centre for Science and Environment, a not for profit organization, recently tested the marketed cosmetics and revealed the presence of mercury in 44 % of fairness creams. Other cosmetics are no less hazarous. The presence of chromium in 50 % and nickel in 43 % of lipstick samples are also detected.

Mercury in any form is highly toxic and potentially dangerous for pregnant woman, foetus and child. Exposure to mercury, even in fairly small amounts, may cause serious health issues. Mercury may have toxic effects on the nervous, digestive and immune system, and on lungs, kidneys and eyes. Mercury released to environment is eaten by fishes. The individuals eating such fishes expose themselves to mercurial toxicities. Realising the toxicity of mercury based products and their environmental impact, worldwide it has been advocated to discontinue the use of mercury based health products. The steps are initiated by various authorities even to replace the mercury based clinical thermometers with digital ones. One can just imagine the health impact of use of such fairness products. The other two heavy metals found in lip sticks are equally hazardous too. Chromium is known to be carcinogenic and the acute ingestion of nickel is known to cause nausea, vomiting, diarrhoea and headache. Nickel too is a known carcinogenic and can cause several harmful effects even deaths. The lipsticks are invariably gets ingested by users.

The advertisement standards council of India too has showed wide spread outrage against the advertisement of fairness products showing darker skin people as inferior. It now proposes for guidelines for such advertisements. Someone once said "We make cosmetics in our factory but we sell hopes in the store". With this hope people continue using them in attempt to improve their appearances. Let's wish the fairness creams would bring more hope than the safety concern!

CHAPTER 68

Anti-High Blood Pressure Medicines

(a) New Hypertension Guideline

Updated Guideline on Hypertension Treatment: A new guideline for prevention, detection, evaluation and management of High Blood Pressure in adults is recently released by American College of Cardiology and American Heart Association. The new definition of hypertension: Systolic BP measurement of 130 mm Hg or higher; or Diastolic BP measurement of 80 mm Hg or higher.

BP Category	Systolic BP		Diastolic BP	Treatment or Follow - up
Normal	<120 mm Hg	And	<80 mm Hg	Evaluate yearly; encourage healthy life style changes.
Elevated	120-129 mm Hg	And	<80 mm Hg	Recommend healthy life style changes and reassess in 3-6 months
Hypertension Stage - 1	130-139 mm Hg	Or	80-89 mm Hg	Assess the 10year risk of heart disease and stroke: • If risk is less than 10%, start with healthy life style recommendations and reassess in 3-6 months; • If the risk is greater than 10% or the patient has known clinical

Contd...

				cardiovascular disease, diabetes mellitus, or chronic kidney disease, recommend life style changes and BP lowering medication (1 medication); reassess in 1 month for effectiveness of medication therapy: • If goal is met after 1 month, reassess in 3-6 months; • If goal is not met after 1 month, consider different medications or titration; • Continue monthly follow-up until control is achieved.
Hypertension Stage 2	≥140 mm Hg	or	≥90 mm Hg	Recommend healthy life style changes and BP lowering medication (2 medications of different classes); reassess in 1 month for effectiveness • If goal is met after 1 month, reassess in 3-6 months • If goal is not met after 1 month, consider different medications or titration • Continue monthly follow – up until control is achieved

(b) Salt Intake - How much is too much?

"High blood pressure (BP) is estimated to cause 7.5 million deaths worldwide which accounts for about 12.8 percent of total all deaths. One in three adults has high BP. Overall prevalence of high BP in adults aged 25 and above was found to be around 40 percent during 2008" the World Health Organization (WHO) reports. India has a slightly lower rate of prevalence compared to global figures but with increasing incidence. In India the blood pressure has increased from 5 percent in 1960s to nearly 12 percent in 1990s and to more than 30 percent in 2008. Cautioning further WHO echoed "High BP increases the risk of heart attacks, strokes and kidney failure. If left uncontrolled it can cause blindness, irregularities in heart beat and heart failure. The risk is higher when the person has diabetes too." People fail to notice the high BP as it does not cause symptoms. High BP is preventable as well as treatable. High BP is defined as systolic BP equal to or above 140 mm of Hg and diastolic BP equal or above 90 mm of Hg, commonly written as 140/90 or higher. In addition to using blood pressure reducing medicines, several strategies have been advocated to control high BP. These include reducing salt intake, eating a balanced diet, avoiding alcohol and smoking, taking regular exercise and maintaining healthy body weight.

Salt provides sodium and chloride. It makes our food tastier. Sodium is a major electrolyte in the extracellular fluid. It plays an important role in nerve conduction and fluid balance in the body. Maintenance of sodium balance depends on kidney function. The body receives sodium from variety of food items like cereals, pulses, vegetables, milk, but the added salt to food is the main concern. Processed and preserved foods like pickles, papads, sauces, ketchups, potato chips etc. contribute to excess salt intake. Sodium makes blood vessels less able to expand and contract and may toughen the heart cells. Besides being risk factors for various cardiovascular issues, the excess sodium intake affects stomach mucosa resulting gastritis and even gastric cancer, greater calcium excretion resulting in loss of bone density. Potassium supplement lowers BP though process is slow. In fact, a balance of sodium and potassium is ideal. Fresh vegetables and fruits are good source of potassium. While excess sodium that we eat due to high salt intake is a concern, no intake of salt at all can prove to be extremely harmful. No salt intake may cause terrible weakness, drowsiness, depression, convulsion and even coma.

Ideally one requires less than 5g of salt per day. Dietary salt intake of less than 3g per day would have significant health impact: health promotion and reduction of many medical costs. A self-care healthy prescription:

- Consume less than one teaspoon of salt a day;
- Avoid junk and process foods;
- Eat more fruits and vegetables;
- Reduce consumption of foods rich in cholesterol, sugar and fat;
- Exercise daily - Even house work, walking, gardening provide good relief;
- Regularly check your BP.

The reducing salt intake helps reducing high blood pressure in salt sensitive persons. This may have little effect on blood pressure of the rest of the population. Nevertheless, since our daily intake of salt vastly exceeds our need for salt cutting, salt intake makes a healthy sense.

(c) Dietary Potassium – Beneficial in Hypertension

The study has shown that that large increases in dietary potassium (above the generally inadequate amounts currently consumed) can significantly lower blood pressure and reduce the occurrence of hypertension and one of its most serious consequences: strokes. An increase in population dietary [potassium] intake of 1.5 [gm/day] could avert over one million deaths from stroke per year on a worldwide scale and is expected to produce overall health benefits by reducing the impact of consequent disabilities.

Modest dietary salt restriction with increasing potassium intake serves as broad spectrum strategy to prevent or control hypertension and decrease cardiovascular morbidity and mortality. Salt intake higher than 8 g/day is considered as a risk factor for hypertension. Dietary potassium intake is recognized as essential public health effort to reduce the rates of hypertension and to prevent kidney disease, stroke and cardiovascular disease. Fruits (Banana, Orange etc.), vegetables (Potatoes, Tomatoes, Beet, Soybeans, Spinach etc.) and milk are rich sources of potassium.

(d) Calcium Channel Blockers Make Dangerous Combination with Most Macrolide Antibiotics

Calcium channel blockers like amlodipine, diltiazem, felodipine, isradipine, nicardipine, nifedipine, nisoldipine and verapamil are primarily used to treat high blood pressure and chest pain caused by coronary artery disease. They are metabolized by cytochrome p4503A4 (CYP3A4) in the liver. The inhibition of the metabolizing enzyme can cause accumulation of dangerously high levels of these high blood pressure treating medicines.

The macrolide group of antibiotics: clarithromycin, erythromycin, azithromycin and telithromycin are used for treatment of a variety of infections in sore throat, sinusitis, acute bronchitis, and community acquired pneumonia. Clarithromycin is also part of regimen used to eradicate *H. pylori* infection in peptic ulcer treatment. The three macrolides: erythromycin, clarithromycin and telithromycin are known potent inhibitor of the metabolizing enzyme CYP3A4. But azithromycin is not a inhibitor of CYP3A4 thus does not show the dangerous effect associated with calcium channel blockers. The grape fruit juice is also known inhibitor of cytochrome p450 3A4. The grape fruit juice has similar effects on calcium channel blockers as clarithromycin or erythromycin.

The various well designed population based studies have reported that amlodipine, diltiazem, felodipine, nifedipine and verapamil when received along with erythromycin or clarithromycin caused hospitalization due to hypotension and acute kidney injury. This even led to deaths. The comparative study of calcium channel blockers and clarithromycin Vs calcium channel blockers and azithromycin showed an increased risk of being hospitalization with acute kidney injury in former. There is an increased absolute risk of 0.22 percent for clarithromycin treated patients and a two-fold relative increase risk. Similarly, the studies have shown higher risks of both being hospitalised with hypotension and dying with clarithromycin treated patients. The risk analysis puts the medicines in the following decreasing order: nifedipine, felodipine and amlodipine. Statistical significant increased risk was not observed in patients treated with diltiazem or verapamil with clarithromycin.

The calcium channel blockers and clarithromycin form a dangerous combination leading to serious adverse effects like hypotension, acute kidney injury and death. The acute kidney injury is attributed to the drop in blood pressure due to excess concentration of calcium channel blockers. This leads to decrease in blood supply to kidney. In our country, the possibility of such combination is high as medicines are freely available even without prescription and there is rampant practice of polypharmacy as well. The clinicians, clinical pharmacists and other pharmacy professionals involved in patient care should take care to avoid such combinations. While the patients are with calcium channel blockers for blood pressure treatment, macrolide antibiotics need to be avoided. If the infection demands the use of macrolide, then azithromycin is a safe choice. The patients too need to be educated not to self medicate with antibiotics in the greater public health interest and to safe-guard themselves from adverse effects of drug-drug interactions.

(e) Healthy Life Style for High Blood Pressure Management

1. Lose weight – Avoid over weight or Obesity;
2. Reduce your salt intake – Reduce your intake of processed and salty foods;
3. Increase your dietary potassium intake – Potassium rich foods include: fresh vegetables and fruits. Ratio of sodium and potassium in diet is important.
4. Restrict Alcohol – If possible should be completely avoided. Beer contains
5. 2-5% and wine 8-10% of alcohol, while brandy, rum and whisky contain much higher concentrations (30-40%);
6. Do Exercise – Exercise regularly to and be physically active to maintain ideal body weight. Adults over the age of 20 years should undertake a minimum of 30-45 minutes of physical activity of moderate intensity (such as brisk walking 5-6 km/hr) 5-6 days of the week. Greater health benefits can be obtained by engaging in physical activity of longer duration or
7. More vigorous intensity such as jogging, running, cycling and swimming.
8. Decrease your fat intake – Butter, ghee, and edible oils are contributors for fat. Minimize the use of processed foods. Ed meat, eggs, organ meats are responsible for contributing cholesterol; and
9. Take fibre rich diets - Dietary fibre delay and retards the absorption of carbohydrates and fats. They also reduce glucose and lipids in bloods; and increase the bulk of stools. Fruits, vegetables, whole grain cereals and pulses are good source of fibre.

CHAPTER 69

Medicine for Lice Treatment

(a) Troublesome Lice

"The child complained of itching on her scalp to her mother. The mother looked at daughter's scalp and found tiny insects all over the head". This is a typical situation of head lice infestation.

Lice are wingless parasites with well developed legs. They spread easily from person to person by body contact. Head lice are the most common lice infestation. Others are body lice and pubic lice. The head louse is scientifically known as *Pediculus humanus capitis*. The lice infestation is also known as pediculosis.

Head lice infest the head and live on the scalp. Female lice lay shiny greyish – white eggs that can be seen as tiny globules firmly stuck to hairs. The eggs are hatched in 5 to 10 days. The newly hatched immature louse resembles an adult and matures within 8 to 9 days. The newly hatched ones are more active than the adults and move around the head. The life span of an adult louse is around one month.

Lice infestation causes severe itching. Intense scratching may break the skin leading often to bacterial infection. Children may hardly notice head lice or may have only vague scalp irritation. The salivary secretion of a louse contains allergic substances that trigger itching. The louse's moth parts pierce the skin and can cause itching too. It takes about 2 to 3 weeks for a person to notice the intense itching.

All family members do require treatment simultaneously.

Presence of live lice must be confirmed before initiating self treatment. Visual inspection of the scalp will verify the presence or absence of head lice or nits (lice eggs). The goal of treatment is to make the infested person free of lice by killing the adult and nymph lice and removing the nits from the person's hair.

Pyrethrins and permethrin are two important lice killing agents. Gamma benzene hexachloride (commonly called Gammaxane) is also very effective. Pyrethrins is generally available in combination with piperonyl butoxide for topical application in the form of solution, shampoos, or gels. It is very safe and can be used on infants, young children and pregnant or lactating women. It has low order of toxicity and adverse effects include irritation, erythema, itching and swelling. Permethrin is available as cream and lotion. Its main adverse effects include itching, stinging and irritation to the scalp. It should not be used on infants younger than 2 years.

All members of the affected household must be treated at the same time, and clothing and bedding should be washed or exposed to air. The hair brushes and combs should also be disinfected. The nit combs can be used to remove lice and nits from the hair.

Here are the general guidelines for appropriate use of the head lice treatment:

- Confirm the presence of live lice on the scalp or hair before initiating self treatment.
- Follow the guidelines as given in the product label or literature. The usual process is to apply the product to clean damp hair and rinse off after 10 minutes.
- Treat all members of the family at the same time.
- Avoid contact with mucous membranes and eyes.
- Avoid physical contact with infested individuals and their belongings like clothing, head gear, brushes, combs and bedding.
- Disinfect combs and brushes by immersing in hot water or using disinfectants.
- Bath and wash the hair often.
- Personal cleanliness is very important. Expose cots, pillow and beddings to direct sun everyday during the treatment period.
- Repeat the treatment in next 7 to 10 days to completely kill the lice.
- Consult health professional, if lice infestation continues even after second treatment.

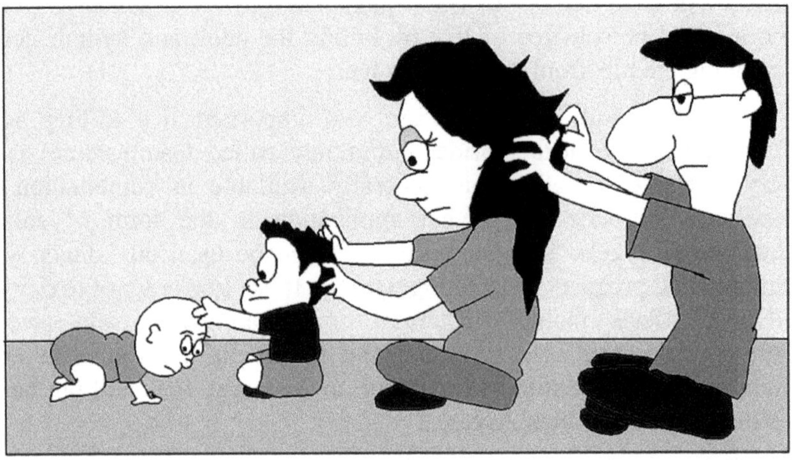

"All family members require treatment simultaneously"

(b) Medicines for Head Lice Treatment

Head lice spread easily from person to person by body contact. Female lice lay shiny greyish-while eggs. These hatched eggs are hatched in 5-10 days. The newly hatched immature louse resembles an adult and matures within 8-9 days. The newly hatched are more active. The life span of an adult louse is around 30 days.

The presence of live lice must be confirmed before initiating the treatment.

Medicine	Instruction of Use (Refer manufacturers' direction for use too)	Issues
Pyrethrins with piperonylbutoxide Shampoo	1. Apply to dry hairs for 10 minutes, then shampoo. 2. Repeat after 7-10 days later.	Allergic reactions may occur rarely. Resistance is also reported.

Contd....

Medicine	Instruction of Use (Refer manufacturers' direction for use too)	Issues
Permethrin1% cream rinse	1. Apply to shampooed, towel dried hairs for 10 minutes and then rinse. 2. Repeat after 7 days.	Pruritis, erythema and edema may occur. Resistance is also reported.
Ivemectin 0.5% lotion	1. Apply to dry hairs and scalp for 10 minutes, then rinse.	Ocular hyperemia, eye irritation, dry skin, burning sensation may occur.
Spinosad 0.9% suspension	1. Apply to dry hairs for 10 minutes, then rinse. 2. Repeat after 7 days if required.	Erythema and irritation of scalp may occur. Irritation in eyes may rarely occur too.
Benzyl alcohol 5% lotion	1. Apply to dry hairs for 10 minutes, then rinse. 2. Repeat after 7 days.	Eye irritation and contact dermatitis may occur.
Malathion 0.5% lotion	1. Apply to dry hairs for 8-12 hours, then shampoo. 2. Repeat after 7 days if necessary.	1. Highly flammable. Do not use a hair dryer or curling iron after applying. 2. Stinging sensation and chemical burns may occur.

Treatment and prevention of transmission are important. The prevention of transmission guidelines are:

- Clean the items that have been in contact with the head of the louse infested person within 24-48 hours;
- Wash the clothing and bed linens in hot water of temperature around 55°C;
- Seal the items (which cannot be washed) in a plastic bag for 48 hours.

CHAPTER 70

Cholesterol Lowering Medicines

(a) Cholesterol lowering medicines

Cholesterol is a fatty wax like substance that circulates through the blood stream. It is an important component of cell membranes, sex hormones, vitamin D, the fluid that coats the lungs, and the protective sheaths around nerve.

The adequate cholesterol level is essential for proper functioning of the body. But the excess cholesterol can clog arteries and increase the risks of cardiovascular diseases. Body obtains cholesterol from two sources: from liver which manufactures and the food we eat. Cholesterol is carried in the blood in protein-lipid package called lipoproteins. The low density lipoprotein (LDL) shuttles cholesterol from the liver to the organs and tissues that require it. The excess unused cholesterol is deposited in the arteries which becomes the risk factors for heart attack and stroke. LDL is called bad cholesterol. High density lipoproteins (HDL) are good cholesterols which shuttle cholesterol back to the liver for recycling.

Statins are potent and effective lipid lowering medicines. They are known to reduce the incidence of fatal and non fatal myocardial infarction, stroke and mortality. It has also proved to have reduced the need for coronary bypass surgery.

Following US FDA's (USA's Drug Regulatory Authority) decision, the Government of India issued safety guidelines to be written on the label of cholesterol lowering statins aiming for judicious use of these medicines. The new potential risks associated with statin use has been identified as: liver injury (though rare), memory loss, risk of diabetes, potential for muscle damage.

Atorvastatin is one of the statins used as adjunct to diet to reduce elevated low density lipoprotein (LDL), total cholesterol, and triglyceride levels. It is contraindicated in persons with active hepatic diseases, pregnant and breast feeding women. Before starting therapy, it is essential to try dietary measures, exercise and cessation of smoking as a means to control cholesterol level.

- Ensure liver function tests before taking statin therapy.

Do not take statins without doctor's advice. Along with medicines follow other methods of reducing cholesterol.

Atorvastatin

- The dose begins at 10 mg daily and may be increased up to 80 mg a day as single dose. Stick to the prescribed dose. Usually the doctor starts with a low dose and then increase depending on requirement.
- Take the tablet at the same time every day with or without food. This is given as once a dosing.
- Do not stop your medicine even if feel better without consulting your doctor.
- If you are pregnant or intending to become pregnant, tell your doctor. The doctor may not prescribe this for you. Do not breast feed as well if you are taking this.
- If you miss a dose, take as soon as you remember. But skip if it is time for the next dose. Do not double your dose at any time.
- Like other medicines, this may also cause side effects. If you experience unusual effects, like muscle pain, tenderness or weakness, immediately report to your doctor.
- Your doctor may ask for periodic liver function tests. Adhere to the instruction.
- Remember the medicine alone does not help. You need to have exercise, weight control and controlled diet. Eat a low cholesterol and low fat diet like cottage cheese, fat free milk, fish, vegetables, egg white. Avoid food with excess fat like: meat, egg yolk, whole milk, cream, butter, cookies, chocolates etc.

Rosuvastatin: Guidelines are similar to that described under Atorvastatin.

(b) Statins for Lowering Cholesterol Level – Using Rationally!

Statins are one of the most prescribed medicines and have been used as weapon for preventing cardiovascular events like heart attacks, strokes etc. The evidence shows that they are effective in reducing the cardiovascular events in persons who are at risk or who have had events earlier but have no benefits (in terms of preventing cardiovascular events) in persons who are at low or no risk. Unfortunately while recommending the use of statins, this aspect is not looked into, but just the elevated cholesterol level. They lower the synthesis of cholesterol. There are several statins currently is use: atorvastatin, fluvastatin, lovastatin, pitavastatin, pravastatin, rosuvastatin, and simvastatin.

The elevated cholesterol level has been viewed as devil and after a laboratory investigation the focus is on reducing the cholesterol level rather than looking the person holistically. It is recommended that total cholesterol should be brought down to below 200 mg/dLand low density lipoprotein (LDL) cholesterol under 100 mg/dL. High cholesterol leads to hardened arteries that can cause heart attack or stroke. But the cholesterol has many vital functions too. The cell membrane is made up of cholesterol. It helps digestion by being part of bile acid production in liver. It is essential for formation of steroids, myelin sheath etc. which are essential for many bodily functions. Everyone needs little bit of cholesterol to work properly. The high density lipoprotein (HDL) is a good cholesterol and at 60 mg/dL or above helps protecting against heart diseases.

Like other medicines, the statins too have their share of concern. They are reported to cause several adverse effects like muscle pain, fatigue, severe life threatening muscle destruction leading to kidney failure (rhabdomyolysis), high blood sugar, liver dysfunction and cognitive impairment. Earlier the country's drug regulatory authority, Drug Controller General, India, has issued instruction to mention the adverse effects that are associated with the use of statins. It is also recommended to have liver function tests prior to recommending statins and thereafter as required. The USFDA removed the warning of the need of routine periodic monitoring of liver enzymes. The routine periodic monitoring of liver enzymes does not found to be effective detecting or preventing serious liver injury.

The life style modification has been proved to be effective in lowering the high cholesterol level in many occasions. Exercises, eating low fat diet, and eating vegetable proteins lower elevated cholesterol and LDL level. Too low fat diet is also not advisable. These non-pharmacological strategies need to be exploited before using statins for controlling elevated cholesterol especially for primary prevention of cardiovascular diseases. However, life-long dietary habits are difficult to change. On the other hand, the statins have proven evidence of preventing the cardiovascular events in persons who are at risk or have a history of events. A judicious use would help the patients and avoid unnecessary exposure to the harmful effects.

CHAPTER 71

Probiotics

(a) Probiotics in Childhood Therapy

Diarrhoea in children is one of the major causes of childhood morbidity and mortality. This is characterized by an abnormally frequent discharge of abnormal volume of semisolid or fluid faecal matter from the bowel. Viral or bacterial intestinal infections, medicines like antibiotics, food or water contaminations, and changes in diet (feed) are common causes of diarrhoea. Whatever may be the reason, the management must have at least three components: rehydration therapy, zinc supplementation and continued feeding.

The increased loss of fluids and electrolytes (sodium, potassium and bicarbonate) that occur during diarrhoea needs to be compensated or replaced by rehydration therapy using Oral Rehydration Salts (ORS). ORS in appropriate quantity helps replacing the loss. However, if the child is sick or severely dehydrated, a medical consultation or attention may be essential. Zinc is an important micronutrient for a child's overall health and development. Zinc is lost in greater quantity during diarrhoea and replacement of lost zinc is essential to help the child recover. A decrease in food intake and decreased nutrient absorption and increased nutrient requirements during diarrhoea may cause malnutrition. Malnutrition can make diarrhoea more severe, more prolonged and more frequent compared to diarrhoea in non-malnourished children. Feeding nutrient rich food (but easily digestible) during diarrhoea is essential.

The antibiotics though not routinely recommended, they are reliably helpful in infectious diarrhoea. In recent times, the probiotics therapy has been recommended as additional therapy for infectious diarrhoea in infants and children. The probiotics therapy has shown to shorten the course of infectious diarrhoea caused by rotavirus and reduce antibiotics associated diarrhoea.

Probiotics are friendly microbes help to maintain the body's delicate microbial balance. Human beings play host to many types and high number of microbes in their body. Most of these bacteria are not harmful and they contribute positively to normal human growth and development. But some of these bacteria can have negative influences. For normal living, it is necessary that the microbial flora be maintained to favour the beneficial bacteria over potentially harmful one.

Probiotics are friendly microbes that help to maintain the body's delicate microbial balance. Curd is a natural probiotic.

Lactobacilli and Bifidobacteria are lactic acid producing bacteria and they constitute a major part of normal intestinal flora. They benefit the host by increasing resistance to new colonization (growth) as well as by protecting against the over growth of all present potentially pathogenic organisms. The use of antimicrobials like antibiotics is the most common cause of disruption of balance of normal microflora. The intestinal microflora provides protection against a broad range of pathogens.

Oral intake of the friendly bacteria (probiotics) helps in normalising the intestinal flora. The lactobacillus bacteria provide protection during diarrhoea by preventing the growth of pathogenic microbes. The various strains of Lactobacillus used: *Lactobacillus acididophilus, Lactic acid bacillus, Lactobacillus casei GG,* Lyophilized *Saccharomyces boulardi* etc. Some of the products available in the market include: Lactflora, Solib, Sporolac.

For centuries, folklore suggested that the fermented dairy products containing live cultures are healthful. Curd is a natural probiotic containing live lactobacillus microbes.

The following precautions need to be taken while taking probiotics:

- Do not drink chlorinated water as chlorine can kill bacteria.
- Avoid antibiotics as they are likely to kill the bacteria present in probiotics products.
- Drink plenty of water. Water helps in flushing out the toxins from the body and help proper adsorption of intestinal flora to gut walls.
- Decrease sugar and processed carbohydrates. These sugars may feed the parasites in intestinal tract and contribute to yeast over growth. This causes imbalance among intestinal flora.

(b) Probiotics in Clinical Use

The probiotics have been known to be beneficial for our health. A recent study report from USA claims that eating probiotics-rich yogurt twice a day for a month can relieve anxiety and stress by reducing activity in the emotional region of the brain. Lets us look at their real status. The probiotics are live, non-pathogenic microorganisms. In USA they are available as dietary supplements and are not approved for any indication. These live microbes usually are bacteria and yeast.

How do they help?

Acetic acid, lactic acid and propionic acid produced by *Lactobacillus* lower intestinal pH and inhibit the growth of pathogenic bacteria like *Escherichia coli* and *Clostridium* spp. The presence of probiotics in the intestinal tract physically and chemically prevents adhesion and colonization of pathogenic bacteria. They may induce or enhance the immune response. These live cultures restore or maintain a healthy microbial flora.

Issues in their Use: The probiotics are not free from adverse effects. They can cause gas, diarrhoea, bloating and hiccups. But they are mild. Infectious complications have also been reported with certain probiotics. Sepsis with *Lactobacillus casei*, fungemia with *S. boulardi* and liver abscess due to *Lactobacillus GG* were reported in highly immunosuppressed and critically ill patients. Antibacterials can inactivate bacteria derived probiotics. Systemic antifungal like fluconazole may inactivate *S. boulardii.* Some of the studies reported that some preparations have been found to contain smaller quantities or different species of organisms to those specified in label.

Sources of probiotics: The curd used by all of us every day is a natural probiotic. But it does not have all types of species. Now the probiotic fortified curd is also available in the market. Probiotics are available as powders, capsules and tablets in medical stores.

Conclusion: The evidence showed that probiotics such as *Lactobacillus* spp. and *Saccharomyces boulardii* are helpful in *Clostridium difficile* infection and antibiotic associated diarrhoea. Though they are believed to be harmless, it is not so. They may cause serious infections in some highly immunosuppressed or critically ill patients. While advising or prescribing probiotics care should be taken: to avoid giving together with antibiotics. The antibiotics kill them. It is necessary wait for the antibiotics course to be over before starting probiotics. The patients are to be advised:

- Check the expiry date before buying.
- Do not freeze acidophilus. Keep the product in a cool, dry place. The refrigerator is preferable.
- Do not drink chlorinated water as chlorine kills bacteria.
- Follow the instruction given on the label of the product.

(c) Friendly Bacteria – for Improved Health!

We have both helpful and harmful bacteria in our body. They are harbored on our skin, gastrointestinal and reproductive tract. The friendly bacteria are natural inhabitant in various parts of our body. The human colon contains friendly bacteria that produce certain vitamins and help digest nutrients. The 5 to 30 feet long gastrointestinal tract of adult individual contains around 100 trillion bacteria with more than 400 diverse species.The friendly bacteria help keeping harmful bacteria in check by competing for food and resources and secreting substances toxic to pathogenic bacteria. There are bacteria in vagina that produce lactic acid and metabolize glycogen secreted by the vaginal epithelium. When enough of these friendly bacteria get destroyed by antibiotic use, the resulting increase in glycogen allows *Candida albicans* to grow causing a yeast infection known as candidiasis. The intestinal epithelium, as it is, acts as physical barrier to the pathogenic bacteria. When the number of good bacteria declines, the pathogenic bacteria can destroy the integrity of the intestinal wall and may cause many illnesses including diarrhea.

These friendly bacteria get disturbed or destroyed often by antibacterial medicines. Though these medicines are intended to kill the harmful ones, they do kill the beneficial bacteria too. The altered intestinal microflora (friendly bacteria) can be substituted or treated with intake of probiotic bacteria. The World Health Organization defines probiotics as “live microorganisms which when administered in adequate amounts confer a health benefit on the host”. They are selected from the strains most beneficial to the intestine: Bacteria from the genera Bifidobacterium & Lactobacillus. These include *Lactobacillus acidophilus, Lactobacillus casei, Lactobacillus plantarum, Bifidobacteriumbifidum, Bifidobacteriumlongum* and *Bifidobacteriuminfantis.* Lactobacilli are available in human and animal mucosal membranes, fermenting and spoiling food.Bifidobacteria belong to the major components of normal intestinal microflora in humans. They appear in the stools a few days after birth.

Our regular foods: curd and yoghurt do contain live bacteria. Curd is a product obtained by souring boiled or pasteurized milk by harmless lactic acid bacteria or other bacterial cultures. The number and type of bacteria in these products vary from home to home. Yoghurt is obtained by lactic acid fermentation of milk *Lactobacillus delbrueckii* and *Streptococcus thermophilus*. Although they have live bacteria and have good nutritional benefits, they do not fall under strict definition of probiotics. The products that are standardized in terms of strain of bacteria, viable count and validated health benefit can only be categorized as probiotics. Now we have curds and yogurts fortified with probiotics. In general probiotics contain one billion live friendly bacteria and are resistant to gastric acid, bile and pancreatic juices, and reach the target site (small and large intestine).

The antibiotics, though not routinely recommended, are reliably helpful in infectious diarrhoea. In recent times, the probiotics therapy has been recommended as additional therapy for infectious diarrhoea in infants and children. The probiotics therapy has shown to shorten the course of infectious diarrhoea caused by rotavirus and reduce antibiotics associated diarrhoea.

While using or taking probiotics one should take note of the following instructions:

- Check the expiry date before buying.
- Do not freeze acidophilus. Keep the product in a cool, dry place. The refrigerator is preferable.
- Avoid antibiotics together. They kill the bacteria. Wait until your antibiotic course is over and then start probiotics.
- Do not drink chlorinated water as chlorine kills bacteria.
- Follow the instruction given on the label of the product.

The Probiotics are essential for good health and beneficial in the treatment and prevention of gastrointestinal diseases!

CHAPTER 72

Others

(a) Aspirin a Day Keeps the Heart Attack Away

Aspirin, a remarkably useful medicine, is valuable in the treatment of many conditions. Earlier we had looked aspirin as pain killer, fever reliever, anti-inflammatory and anti-rheumatic medicine. It makes the blood less able to clot and this property has been used to discover the usefulness of aspirin in preventing and management of cardiac disorders.

Like other organs of the body, heart too needs regular blood supply for healthy functioning. The bulk of the blood is supplied by the coronary arteries. Any damage to these important blood vessels can cause a reduction of blood supply (including oxygen and other nutrients) to specific areas of heart muscles. Some arteries of the heart often completely or severely blocked depriving oxygen and nutrient supply to heart muscles. Medically this condition is called myocardial infraction and in general term heart attack. The word heart attack is frightening and emergency condition. The death rate is high. On an average: half of deaths occur in the first few hours after the symptoms begin to appear. A prompt medical attention can save life.

A blood clot is the most common cause of a blocked coronary artery. Aspirin prevents heart attack by interfering with the clotting mechanisms in which blood platelets clump together to form clots. It inhibits irreversibly platelet cyclooxygenase responsible for synthesis of thromboxane A_2. This thromboxane A_2 causes platelet aggregation. Thus aspirin inhibits the formation of blood clots in the arteries and does not reverse atherosclerosis (narrowing of arteries) in the coronary arteries. Aspirin reduces the risk of death and the risk of second heart attack by 15 to 30 percent.

The recommended dose of aspirin for preventing heart attack is much less than the dose required for other uses. Often this reduced dose is called a baby aspirin. Higher dose must be avoided as it may have opposite effect – formation of blood clots. The dose of 75 to 100 mg daily is suggested as prophylactic dose for preventing heart attack or stroke. For long-term management of already heart attack patients, a dose of 75 to 150 mg daily is recommended. If immediate effect is required as in the initial treatment of heart attack a loading dose of 150 to 300 mg be given preferably by dispersing in water or swallowed after chewing. On shifting the patient to the medical care centre this fact needs to be told to the treating doctor (patient has already been given aspirin).

Avoid in the last three months of pregnancy as it may prolong pregnancy and labour besides causing bleeding.

Any male or female with a family history of heart attack and high cholesterol levels, inactive life style, diabetes and smoking cigarettes; postmenopausal women with one or more risk factors for heart disease are prime candidates for using aspirin as a preventive measure. The regular prophylaxis use of aspirin is probably not justified by healthy individuals.

Here are few practical tips for using aspirin safely and effectively:

- Discuss with your doctor before using aspirin as prophylactic therapy for preventing heart attack and stroke. Your doctor will check the risk factors.
- If used in the initial treatment of heart attack, this should be informed to treating doctor immediately or on arrival to medical care centre.
- Often your doctor prescribes enteric-coated aspirin tablets to prevent gastric ill effects associated with its use. Do not take gastric antacids immediately after swallowing these enteric – coated products. Do not split them too.
- Avoid use of this medicine during last three months of pregnancy. It can prolong pregnancy and labour. It can cause bleeding before and after delivery.
- Avoid use of aspirin if individual is sensitive or allergic to aspirin, has asthma, problem of wound healing including bleeding ulcers. Your doctor may suggest an alternative to aspirin.

- Inform your doctor or pharmacist, if you experience any side or undesirable effects.

Some studies have also suggested the usefulness of aspirin in reducing the risk of lung, colon and breast cancer. But conclusive evidence are lacking.

(b) Aspirin to Prevent Coronary Heart Diseases – Is Routine Use Justified?

Cardiovascular disease (CVD) is the leading cause of deaths and disability worldwide. The percentage of premature deaths due to CVD ranges from 4% in developed countries to as high as 42% in economically poor countries. Of the various forms of CVD, the coronary heart disease (CHD) and cerebrovascular disease (stroke) are the leading contributors for mortality due to CVD. Low dose aspirin is routinely used to prevent cardiovascular events. Aspirin acts by preventing aggregation of platelets which may cause clots. Platelets combine with the cholesterol in the arterial wall to form a clot and block the heart artery. The blockage leads to heart attack. Aspirin prevents the clot formation due to its anti-platelet activity.

The recent study reported in the American Heart Association's Journal "Arteriosclerosis, Thrombosis, and Vascular Biology′ following a 10 years observation "Genetic variation may modify the cardiovascular benefit of aspirin even harming some patients". This raises a concern of aspirin's routine use. COMT is a key enzyme in the metabolism of catecholamines: epinephrine, norepinephrine, and dopamine. There are three variants of COMT: enzyme's low activity methionine form (met/mets), the enzyme's high activity valine form (val/vals) and intermediate activity (val/met) with in between high and low activities. Individuals with highactivity valine form have been shown to have lower levels of catecholamines compared to individuals with methionine form. The 23 percent of the women who were 'val/vals' were naturally protected against incident cardiovascular disease but when women with the similar genetic type were allocated to aspirin, this natural protection was eliminated. Further investigation shown that val/val women who were randomly assigned to aspirin had more cardiovascular events than the val/vals who were assigned to placebo. On the other hand, among the 28 percent of met – women there were fewer cardiovascular events when assigned to aspirin compared to placebo. The study indicates that the genetic variation has profound influence on aspirin's activity.

USFDA, perhaps the strongest drug regulatory authority in the world, has declined the Bayer AG Company's request for permission to make a change in the labelling that would have allowed the company to market aspirin as preventive therapy for people who have no heart problems. The regulator warns "Benefits of aspirin outweighs the risks in cases where people have already experienced stroke or heart attacks".

While the studies have confirmed the usefulness of aspirin in primary prevention of cardiovascular events, its use is not free of risks. Aspirin can produce serious adverse effects. The aspirin is known to increase the incidence of gastrointestinal bleeding and haemorrhagic stroke. The present findings further increase the risk of using aspirin at least in some group of people (genetically variant). The physicians and the practicing pharmacists should refrain from routine use of aspirin for preventing CVD but restrict to those who are with moderate or high risk. Its combination with other platelet aggregation inhibitors should not be used routinely.

(c) Word of Caution for Aspirin Poppers!

The daily use of aspirin is not right for everyone! The US regulatory authority warns. Aspirin has been in clinical practice as gold standard for preventing heart attack and other cardiovascular events. The recent research finding shows that in some patients it is just reverse. Instead of protecting the patients it makes them more vulnerable for cardiac events.

Cardiovascular disease (CVD) is the leading cause of deaths and disability worldwide. The percentage of premature deaths due to CVD ranges from 4% in developed countries to as high as 42% in economically poor countries. Of the various forms of CVD, the coronary heart disease (CHD) and cerebrovascular disease (stroke) are the leading contributors for mortality due to CVD. Low dose aspirin is routinely used to prevent cardiovascular events. Aspirin acts by preventing aggregation of platelets which may cause clots. Platelets combine with the cholesterol in the arterial wall to form a clot and block the heart artery. The blockage leads to heart attack. Aspirin prevents the clot formation due to its anti-platelet activity. In such situation aspirin continues to be used for years together.

The recent study reported in the American Heart Association's Journal "*Arteriosclerosis, Thrombosis, and Vascular Biology'* following a 10 years observation "Genetic variation may modify the cardiovascular benefit of aspirin even harming some patients". This raises a concern of aspirin's routine use. COMT is a key enzyme in the metabolism of catecholamines: epinephrine, norepinephrine, and dopamine. There are three variants of COMT: enzyme's low activity methionine form (met/mets), the enzyme's high activity valine form (val/vals) and intermediate activity (val/met) with in between high and low activities. Individuals with high activity valine form have been shown to have lower levels of catecholamines compared to individuals with methionine form. The 23 percent of the women who were 'val/vals' were naturally protected against incident cardiovascular disease but when women with the similar genetic type were allocated to aspirin, this natural protection was eliminated. Further investigation shown that val/val women who were randomly assigned to aspirin had more cardiovascular events than the val/vals who were assigned to placebo. On the other hand, among the 28 percent of met – women there were fewer cardiovascular events when assigned to aspirin compared to placebo. The study indicates that the genetic variation has profound influence on aspirin's activity.

USFDA, perhaps the strongest drug regulatory authority in the world, has declined the Bayer AG Company's request for permission to make a change in the labelling that would have allowed the company to market aspirin as preventive therapy for people who have no heart problems. The regulator warns "Benefits of aspirin outweighs the risks in cases where people have already experienced stroke or heart attacks". Remember, there may be a benefit to daily aspirin use for you if you have some kind of heart or blood vessel disease, or if you have evidence of poor blood flow to the brain. However, the risks of long-term aspirin use may be greater than the benefits if there are no signs of, or risk factors for heart or blood vessel disease.

While the studies have confirmed the usefulness of aspirin in primary prevention of cardiovascular events, its use is not free of risks. Aspirin can produce serious adverse effects. The aspirin is known to increase the incidence of gastrointestinal bleeding and haemorrhagic stroke. The present findings further confirm the risk of using aspirin at least in some group of people (genetically variant). The proverb 'Aspirin a day keeps the heart attack away' is now under scanner. Till more evidence arises, it is advisable to restrict the regular use of aspirin only to the patients who are at risk!

(d) Clopidogrel

Clopidogrel, an antiplatelet medicine, has been recommended either alone or with aspirin to prevent serious or life threatening problems with the heart and blood vessels in people who have had a stroke, heart attack, or severe chest pain and peripheral arterial disease. The latest US FDA review finds that long-term use of this blood-thinning drug does not increase or decrease the overall risk of death in patients with, or at risk for, heart disease.

Analysis suggests that long term (>12 months) dual antiplatelet therapy [clopidogrel + aspirin] does not appear to change the overall risk of death when compared to short term (<6 months) clopidogrel and aspirin, or aspirin alone. The review does not suggest that clopidogrel increases the risk of cancer or death from cancer.

Availability and Dose: Oral Tablet of 75 mg or 300 mg is to be taken once a day preferably at the same time of the day before or after meals.

Caution: Clopidogrel increases the risk of bleeding especially if taken in combination with aspirin, NSAIDs like ibuprofen and naproxen, warfarin, selective serotonin reuptake inhibitors and serotonin norepinephrine reuptake inhibitors. The medicine has to be stopped before dental procedures.

Contraindicated in pregnancy or breast feeding, liver and kidney dysfunction.

Adverse effects: The most frequent adverse effects are bruising and bleeding, such as nose bleeds or less commonly, blood in the urine or faeces. Diarrhoea and abdominal pain are also fairly common. Rare adverse effects include nausea, vomiting, headache, dizziness, constipation, rash, itching, sore throat, fever, and shortness of breath.

(e) Power of Antioxidants

The vast majority of complex life requires oxygen for its existence. Without oxygen, life is unthinkable. But oxygen is a highly reactive molecule that damage living organisms including humans by producing reactive oxygen species. The reactive oxygen species (oxidants) produced in the cells includes free radicals beside others. These oxidants damage cellular components such as DNA, proteins and lipids. Damage to DNA can cause mutations and possibly cancer while damage to proteins leads to enzyme inhibition, denaturation and protein degradation. Fortunately the life contains a complex net work of multiple types of antioxidants to prevent oxidative damage to cells.

Low levels of antioxidant molecules cause oxidative stress and damage or kill cells. Oxidative stress has been implicated in the pathogenesis of many human diseases and use of antioxidants has been recommended.

Antioxidants are molecules that slow or prevent oxidation. They reduce, neutralise, and prevent damage done to the body by free radicals. The damage caused by free radicals includes deterioration of bones, joints, and connective tissues; wearing of organs; the decline of immune systems and advancement of visible effects of aging. They have been found to have benefit as defence against the risk of developing certain illness and diseases. Even they are conceptualized as insurance against visible effects of aging.

There are several enzyme systems in the body that scavenge free radicals. The most important micronutrient antioxidants are Vitamin E, Beta Carotene, Vitamin C, Selenium and Lycopene. The body can not manufacture these micronutrients and they must be supplied in the diet or through other supplementation.

Though the role of antioxidants have been advocated as possible treatment for neurodegenerative diseases such as Alzheimer's disease, Parkinson's disease, but their usefulness has no conclusive evidence. Similar is the case of effects of antioxidants in aging.

Oxidation of low density lipoprotein in the blood contributes to heart disease and accordingly the vitamin E supplementation was recommended to lower the risk of developing heart disease. But the recent study proved that there is no significant effect of vitamin E in over all deaths or on deaths due to heart disease.

Pre-eclampsia (eclampsia means sudden fits) can occur during pregnancy when women have high blood pressure and protein in urine often leading to serious complications including mortality. Supplementation of antioxidants such as Vitamin C, Vitamin E, Selenium and lycopene prevent pre-eclampsia.

Age related muscular degeneration affect central area of the retina (back of the eye). The retina can deteriorate with age and some people get lesions that can lead to central vision. The progression of disease may be slowed down in people who eat a diet rich in antioxidant vitamins and minerals.

Fruits and vegetables are good sources of anti-oxidants.

They have no role in preventing gastrointestinal cancer. The study even proved that they increase mortality.

These antioxidants have been marketed as medicines, nutraceuticals or as dietary supplements.

The diets rich in fruit and vegetables, which are high in antioxidants, promote health and reduce the effects of aging, reduce the risk of cancer, heart disease and some neurological diseases. However, the usefulness of antioxidants' supplementation has no conclusive evidence. It is preferable to eat plenty of fruits and vegetables with high antioxidant contents to get benefit from these micronutrients tackling the ill effects of free radicals. Vitamin E is present in nuts, seeds, vegetables and fish oils, whole grains, fortified cereals and apricot. Vitamin C is plenty in citrus fruits and juices, green peppers, cabbage, spinach etc. Beta –carotene is available in liver, egg yolk, milk, butter, spinach, carrots etc. Lycopene is found in tomato and tomato products, pink grape fruits, water melon.

There is one more reason for preferring fruits and vegetables as source of antioxidants. Once antioxidant supplements are thought to be harmless, but there is potential for interaction and toxicity. In the normal concentration found in the body, vitamin C and beta-carotene are antioxidants; but at higher concentrations they are pro-oxidants and thus harmful.

(f) Steroids in COPD Management

Chronic Obstructive Pulmonary Disease (COPD), a new terminology, is now widely accepted for emphysema or chronic bronchitis or both. COPD has become one of the major causes of morbidity and mortality. Worldwide more than 3 million people died due to COPD in 2005 which accounts to 5 % of all deaths globally in 2005. Though no reliable data is available, the various study reported the prevalence of COPD in India is slightly more than 4%. Being a chronic and progressive disease process, it causes a huge economic burden to the patients and the health system as well. Though the primary cause of COPD is tobacco smoke, the indoor and outdoor environmental pollution are also risk factors.

The common symptoms include breathlessness, coughing and phlegm. The acute condition with worsening of patients' respiratory situation often requires hospitalization and medical intervention. In mild COPD, the shortness of breath may occur only with exertion. The most common medicine interventions include the use of bronchodilator (s) and steroids. The bronchodilators widen the tubes of lungs and the steroid helps in controlling the underlying inflammation in the lungs. The inhaled bronchodilators improve symptoms, decrease exacerbations and improve quality of life. The inhaled and systemic steroids have beneficial effects in acute exacerbation of COPD. Though the present article is not intended to discuss the pros and cons of various treatment options, the following recent appeared evidences would serve as guide for promoting rational therapy:

- A 7 to 14 days treatment with oral glucocorticoid (prednisone / prednisolone) is recommended for acute exacerbated COPD.This is known to shorten the recovery time and hospitalization duration, improve lung function and blood oxygen levels, and reduces the risk of treatment failure and a recurrent exacerbation in short term. The recent study reports that a **short five day course of glucocorticoid therapy for acute COPD exacerbation works equally as 14 days course for most patients**. This finding enables the healthcare providers to minimize steroid exposure and reduce the steroid related harms in patients. Stopping the medicine is as important as starting it. The oral corticosteroids are ineffective and are not recommended in stable COPD.

- The combined inhalation treatment with inhaled steroid and long acting beta agonist is often used. The combined treatment (Budesonide + Formoterol; Fluticasone + Salmeterol) is more effective than long acting beta agonist [LOBA] alone in improving health related quality of life. The recent study showed that **there is increased risk of pneumonia with combined inhalers from around 3 per 100 people per year on LOBA to 4 per 100 per year on combined inhalers. Approximately every 17 people treated with combined inhaler, one extra person may get pneumonia (compared to placebo)**. There is also increased risk of candidiasis. Guiding the patients on appropriate use of inhalers and instructing to wash the mouth after each inhalation would reduce the chances of fungal infection.

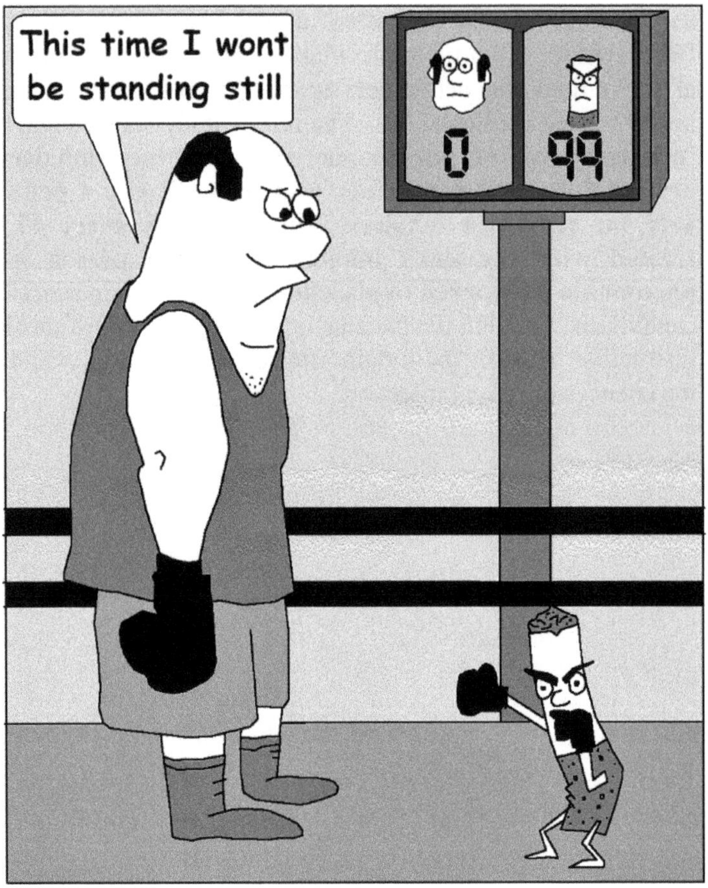

"Its never too late to quit smoking"

(g) Nicotine Replacement Medicines

"Tobacco is deadly in any form or disguise," says an advertisement released on World No Tobacco Day, 31st May 2006. Statutory warning in cigarette packets writes, "Smoking is injurious to health". Many continue to ignore such alarms. Tobacco is smoked in the form of manufactured cigarettes. Bidi, chulta (cigar), chillum, and hookah are the indigenous form of smoking. Smoking is one of the most serious health hazards.

Everyday over 2200 people die due to tobacco use in our country. Over 55,000 young people take to smoking every year. Smoking killed nearly five million people worldwide in 2000 of which one-third of the reported deaths were from India.

The principal ingredients consumed during smoking of tobacco include nicotine, tar and carbon monoxide. It causes an increased risk of cardiovascular disease such as coronary heart disease and stroke, lung and other forms of cancer, and respiratory diseases such as chronic bronchitis. Smoking diminishes fertility in women and increases the risk of ectopic pregnancy, miscarriage, preterm birth, preclampsia, and stillbirth. The combination of smoking and oral contraceptive is dangerous.

Nicotine is a toxic and dependence producing psychotropic substance. A few drops of pure nicotine, weighing around 60 mg, on the tongue can kill a healthy adult. Cigarettes usually contain 0.5-2.0 mg of nicotine depending upon brand. Nicotine dependence is the central factor in the continuation of smoking behaviour.

Though many smokers give up through strong determination, motivation and encouragement; nicotine replacement therapy is an important part of treatment process for some patients. When people quit smoking health risk decreases rapidly. Unfortunately nicotine dependence is very strong, it is difficult to quit smoking permanently. Irritability, anxiety, decreased heart rate, increased appetite, food cravings, restlessness and difficulty in concentrating are the common withdrawal signs and symptoms of giving up smoking (nicotine withdrawal).

It is never too late to quit smoking. "Cigarette – Fire at one end and the Fool at the other."

Nicotine replacement medicines supply the smokers (and other tobacco users) with nicotine from other sources. Although still harmful, they provide a cleaner form of nicotine unlike tobacco. These avoid the exposure to other thousands poisons like carbon monoxide, tar etc., that are found in burning tobacco. In this way, the withdrawal effect of not smoking is less severe. As body adjusts to not smoking, the use of these medicines is decreased gradually over few weeks. Finally use is stopped altogether.

The most common form of nicotine replacement medicine is available as flavoured chewing gum or a skin patch. It is used for up to 12-20 weeks as part of supervised step in smoking cessation programme. Like other medicines, it is also to be used appropriately to maximise benefits while minimising the risk associated with its use. It is not suitable for use during pregnancy and breast-feeding. Smoking needs to be avoided during using these medicines as combination may cause overdosing of nicotine. The chewing gum tablets and skin patches come with directions for use. The user needs to understand the proper use of these medicines. Here are the usual guidelines one needs to adhere:

While using chewing gum tablets:

- Chew one piece of gum very slowly when you have an urge to smoke. Chewing about 30 minutes will provide full dose of nicotine.
- Do not chew too fast, do not use more than one piece at a time and do not chew too often. They may cause overdosing.
- Gradually reduce the number of pieces of gum you chew everyday as your urge to smoking reduces.
- More than 30 pieces is not advisable (chances of overdosing).
- Do not use longer than 6 months (may cause physical dependence).
- Keep away from children.

While using skin patches:

- Clean your hands.
- Clean and dry the area of application completely. Do not use over bruised or damaged skin or over skin folds.
- Remove the patch from package taking care not to tear or cut the system.
- Remove the protective liner and firmly press against the skin site for about 10 seconds. Rub the edges to seal.
- Rinse your hand with plain water after you have finished applying patch. Using soap during washing may increase penetrability of nicotine to your body.
- Wear for full periods as instructed in product information inserts or as directed by your doctor (not more than 24 hours).

- Remove at the end of use and fold the use system in half with adhesive layer together to prevent its further use and then dispose off.
- For repeated use, apply the new patch to a new site preferably at the same time each day.

It is never too late to quit smoking. Visit your doctor and consult him/her to know more on smoking cessation aids or therapy.

(h) Worrisome Worms

"Child started crying in the night and complained of itching around the anus. The mother looked at the site and found white tiny thread like worms around anus". This is the typical symptom of pinworm infection.

The pinworms are the most common parasite in children in tropical areas. They are scientifically known as *Enterobius vermicularis.* They are around 1 cm long and too known threadworms. The infection is called enterobiasis.

The most common method of transmission of pinworms is the direct anus to mouth transfer of eggs when children use contaminated fingers to handle and take food. Re-infection may readily occur because eggs are often found under the fingernails of infected children who have scratched the anal area. The transfer of eggs may also occur from perianal area of an infected individual to bedding, clothing, toys etc., where eggs are picked up by new hosts, introduced into the mouth and swallowed. Eggs dislodged from perianal area into the environment may survive for as long as 3 weeks and cab inhaled or swallowed. The eggs hatch releasing the larvae into the small intestine. After few weeks the mature female worms migrate to the anal area and discharge eggs and continue the cycle.

The children carrying pinworm infection often have no symptoms. The first symptom of worm infection is the presence of worms in the stool. But is difficult to detect in the stool. However, the most common symptom is the feeling of itching around the anus and the children have the tendency to continuously scratch the area. Though these parasites rarely cause any harm, the pinworm infection may cause vaginal itching and irritation. In rare cases, appendicitis may be caused by pinworms blocking the appendix. Too much scratching to relieve the itching may cause small ulcers around the anus often leading to secondary bacterial infection.

All family members require simultaneous treatment to prevent spreading of infection from one to the other.

The diagnosis of pinworm infection is made by finding the worms. The visual inspection of child's anal area with a flashlight about 1-2 hours after the child has been put to sleep at night. The worms are visible to the naked eye. The pinworm infection may be self-limiting but the infection is uncomfortable.

The treatment aims to eradicate pinworms from the patient and other members of the household, thereby preventing re-infection. All household members should be treated concurrently with a single dose of mebendazole, albendazole or pyrantel. Since re-infection readily occurs, at least one more dose is advised 2-4 weeks later. Piperazine too is effective but needs to be taken regularly for at least seven days.

Medicine	Availability	Dose
Albendazole	Chewable tablets	Adult and child over 2 years: 400 mg. Child 12 months to 2 years: 200 mg.
Mebendazole	Chewable tablets	Adult and child over 2 years: 100 mg. Second dose after 2- 3 weeks
Pyrantel	Chewable tablets and suspension	Dose is weight dependent. 10 mg/kg body weight as single dose. Second dose after 2-4 weeks.

The above medicines are useful for other intestinal worms infections too, but doses are different.

The medicines by themselves are not enough to get rid of pinworm infections. Personal, family and public hygiene are equally important. Here are few guidelines:

- All family members must take medicines because re-infection can spread from one family member to the other.
- Do not self medicate under the following conditions: if you have liver disease, anaemia or pregnancy; or you are breast-feeding; in children under 2 years of age.
- If you experience any other side effects, inform your doctor or pharmacist. The side effects for these medicines are usually not serious.
- Strict hygiene is essential to prevent spreading of infections. Washing of hands and buttock after each passing of motion is a must.
- Toilet should be frequently disinfected.

- All under garments, nightclothes and bed linens should be washed/or cleaned daily until the patient is free of worms.
- The infected child should wear tight diapers or pants while sleeping to keep him or her off from scratching the anus.

(i) Steam Inhalation in Acute Respiratory Tract Infection!

Acute Respiratory Tract infections are common conditions often treated at primary care levels. The common symptoms are: unwell feeling, sleep disturbances, fever, interference with normal activities, sore throat, cough, short of breath, facial or sinus pain, earache, and running or blocked nose. In addition to advice of taking common analgesics and antipyretics like paracetamol, the steam inhalation too commonly advised. The use of antibiotics is always controversial as some times these infections are caused by viruses.

Some of the symptoms are attributed to congestion arising from the swelling of the membranes and thickened mucous in the nose. The steam inhalation is believed to help the patient by lightening the respiratory tract secretions and relieving the symptoms of respiratory distress. Breathing in steam from a bowl or jug is steam inhalation. The steam inhalation is commonly practiced by holding head under a towel over a bowl of very hot water. It is the inhalation of humidified air. There are no enough studies conducted to test the efficacy of steam inhalation in providing relief in acute respiratory tract infection. Even there is no consistent benefit in the treatment of common cold. Never the less, this steam inhalation is common and inexpensive therapy.

There have been conflicting reports on the usefulness of steam inhalation in acute respiratory tract infections. While some reports confirmed the symptomatic relief, the others showed no objective improvement in outcome measures such as viral shedding or viral titres in nasal washings. The common technique of steam inhalation is always associated with injury like scalding or steam burn. This risk of injury is much higher in young children as they do not understand the safety aspects often burning their faces. Patients or parents need to be advised on the risk involved and take precautions to avoid injury. It is often said "Sit in the bath room with a hot shower running", a safe mode of steam inhalation therapy.

(j) Fighting Bird Flu with Tamiflu

The deadly H5N1 bird flu virus continues resurfacing. Fortunately, no human bird flu is detected so far though some of persons showing bird flu symptoms have been quarantined and treated with Tamiflu, the most effective antiviral against avian influenza.

Household or close family contacts of strongly suspected or confirmed H5N1 patient are at high risk and persons handling sick animals or decontaminating the affected environments including animal disposal, individuals with unprotected and very close direct exposure to sick or dead animals infected with H5N1 virus are at moderate risk of getting infected. Of all influenza A virus that circulate in birds, H5N1 virus is most deadly and caused by far the greatest number of human cases of very serious diseases and the greatest number of deaths.

The infection of bird flu is suspected when flu like symptoms like fever, cold, body aches, running nose and/or eyes, loss of appetite, when the person is recently in contact with the poultry in bird flu affected area. When such symptoms appear, immediate medical attention is necessary. Family members taking care of the infected person should protect themselves by wearing mask, cleaning all the surfaces that come in contact with hands or secretions of the patients with soap, Lysol (antiseptic) etc. Patients should restrict movement. It would prevent further spreading of infection.

Tamiflu is the brand name of the medicine "Oseltamivir". This is a prescription only medicine known as the first choice in treating avian influenza. The recommended dose for adults is 75 mg orally twice daily for 5 days beginning within 2 days of symptom onset. Patient vomiting within one hour of ingestion may be given another one capsule of 75 mg. The children dose is weight dependent. One needs to consult doctor for the exact dose for children. The dosage adjustment is necessary in renal impaired patients.

Prophylaxis antiviral treatment is necessary in high or moderate risk groups. Administration of Oseltamivir should begin as soon as possible after the exposure status is known and be used continuously for 7 to 10 days after last known exposure. The adult recommended dose for prophylaxis is 75 mg once a day for 7 to 10 days. Children require dose based on their weight.

Complete the course of medicine even if you feel better.

Nausea and vomiting are the two common adverse effects reported. These can be avoided by taking medicine with/after food or milk.

The medicine seems to be not available for sale in the market. But some pharmaceutical companies have assured government to supply the required quantity of medicines even with short notice. The companies are ready with the generic version of Tamiflu.

The General Guidelines for safe and effective use of Oseltamivir:

- Contact your doctor as soon as symptoms appear.
- Avoid self medication.
- Complete the full 5 day's course even if you feel better.
- Take medicine with food or milk to avoid side effects like nausea and vomiting. This can be taken without meals too.
- If a dose is missed, take it as soon as possible. But skip the dose if the next dose is within 2 hours. Do not double your dose.
- Inform your doctor if you have kidney problem. Dose adjustment may be necessary.

(k) Chikungunya Treating Medicine

"As many as 121 districts of Tamil Nadu, Karnataka, Maharastra, Madhya Pradesh, Gujarat and Kerala have been affected by the Chikungunya disease. A total of 9,74,541 cases have been reported." Health Minister said in parliament on 26th July 2006. It is like a situation of health emergency.

Though you might feel quite OK last night, find painful in the morning, unable to get up from the bed. One would have a feeling of somebody breaking his/her bones, wrists and hands. Muscles become so hard that one cannot do anything. One experiences these symptoms if affected by Chikungunya. It has flu like symptoms such as severe headache, chills, fevers, joint pains, nausea, vomiting etc. Some people may have bleeding from nose or gums. In severe cases, respiratory failure, cardiovascular decompensation (not balancing the functional or structural defects), or meningoencephalitis may occur.

Chikungunya is a rare form of viral fever caused by an alphavirus. This is spread through mosquito bites by the *Aedes aegypti* mosquitoes in human to human. The disease was first described in Tanzania, an African State in as early as 1952. The outbreak of the disease in India is reported in early 2006. The incubation period is about one to twelve days after mosquito biting. Unfortunately, there is no cure or treatment for Chikungunya and the main problem with this viral fever is the after effects. The fever may subside within three to five days but the joint pains persist for months.

The disease is self-limiting and resolves with time, but needs supportive medical care with anti-inflammatory and analgesic medicines. Paracetamol is used for treating fever and anti-inflammatory drugs like Aspirin, Ibuprofen, Diclofenac, Naproxen etc., used for treating knee or joint pain. The chloroquine phosphate is also recommended for acute joint symptoms. Doxycycline or tetracycline for 5 to 7 days can also be explored as prophylactic.

Prevent mosquito breeding to protect yourself from mosquito transmitted diseases.

As no medicine is absolutely safe without any side or toxic effects, it is essential that the patients use them with caution and take advises of doctors or pharmacists. Few common problems associated with the above medicines: paracetamol with liver toxicity, aspirin with gastrointestinal upset and even bleeding, ibuprofen with bronchial asthma, diclofenac with gastric irritation, naproxen with gastric irritation and so on. Aspirin is not recommended for children. The asthma patients should avoid non-steroidal anti-inflammatory agents like ibuprofen. Alcoholic patients should be careful while taking paracetamol as alcohol increases the chances of liver toxicity. Chloroquine is usually used in malaria. It may cause blurred vision and should be used with caution in patients with retinal or visual problems.

Though Chikungunya is not a deadly disease, but some deaths were reported from some parts of the country. It is thought because of inappropriate use of the medicines. This is highly infectious and disabling. As no cure is available, it is best to take preventive steps. Unfortunately there is no vaccine. The only and perhaps best option available is to maintain cleanliness. Removal of all open containers with stagnant water in and around our residence would prevent mosquito breeding, the transmitter of disease. The adult mosquitoes can be killed through spraying of insecticides. Keep the surroundings clean with no stagnation of water to prevent the mosquitos' transmitted diseases like Malaria, Filaria and Chikungunya.

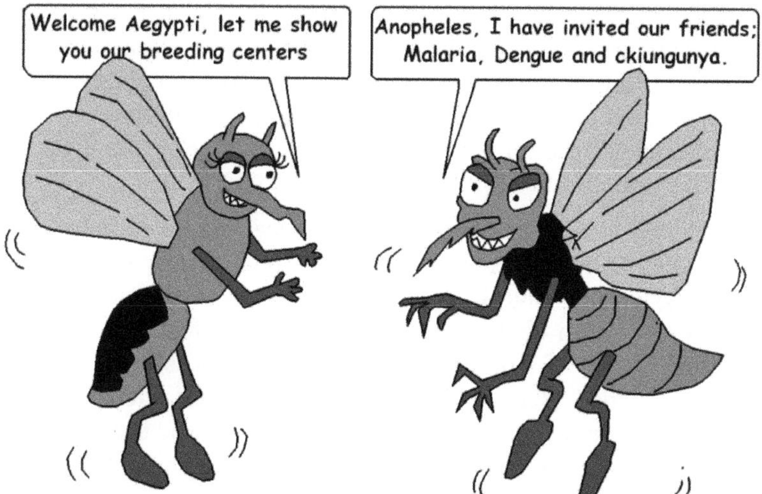
Welcome Aegypti, let me show you our breeding centers
Anopheles, I have invited our friends; Malaria, Dengue and ckiungunya.

"Prevent the breeding of mosquitoes to stop spreading of mosquito transmitted diseases"

(I) Darker Side of Your Antibacterial Toilet Soaps!

Hand washing is not only part of our cultural habit and religious faith, but has great importance in preventing infections and illness. Microorganisms are present everywhere and we often use toilet soaps with antibacterial agents in order to remove them from our body including hands. We believe, perhaps more because of influence from advertisement, that the antibacterial soaps are more effective and better than ordinary soap. It is just another myth. The United States Food and Drugs Administration (USFDA) has just confirmed that antibacterial soaps and liquid washes are no better than ordinary soap and water. It cautioned "long term use of these products are harmful too". USFDA, world's most effective regulatory agency, is mandated to protect and promote public health in USA.

The antibacterial soaps and washes contain chemicals like triclosan and triclocarbon. Triclosan is used in liquid soap and triclocarbon in toilet soap. They are used along with water and rinsed off after use. They are promoted for being superior to non-bacterial washes in preventing human illness or reducing illness. Manufacturers of these products failed to provide evidence of their superiority. Triclosan, a synthetic antimicrobial, is introduced into use as an ingredient of disinfectant hand wash lotions for hospital staff. Now this is found in almost all our personal products: cosmetics, tooth pastes, household cleansers, detergents, sports clothing and kitchen utensils. But has been under scanner of the authorities for its reported adverse effects.

The animal studies show that this chemical enhances the growth of breast cancer cells, adversely affect the functioning of muscles and hormone system, damage liver and possibly cause of emergence liver cancer on long term contact. While the animal effects may not be the complete evidence of similar ill effects in humans, but definitely risks cannot be excluded. Because of their wide and unrestricted use, they are now detected even in the urine of pregnant women. The tested cord blood samples too show the presence of triclosan threatening their entry to foetus too. A recent study by the Toxic Links (India) found the presence of this compound in personal care products. Of the eleven samples of liquid soaps, one sample was found to have Triclosan concentration of

3068 ppm (0.3068%), higher than the BIS standards. In case of tooth pastes, out of eleven samples, four samples contained high concentration of the chemical than as prescribed by BIS standards of 0.3 %. The unrestricted and rampant use of these chemicals give rise to microbial resistance too. The irresponsible way of promoting bacterial resistance with proliferation of more super bugs! The microbial resistance has been recognised as one of the biggest threat human kind is currently facing.

Triclosan Containing Antiseptic Products Not Safe for Use

The US Food and Drug Administration (FDA) has ruled that 24 active ingredients used for preparing OTC healthcare antiseptics are not recognised as safe and effective. The FDA wants to evaluate them as new drugs. Triclosan is one of these 24 ingredients most frequently used in India. Wide variety of products, available in Indian market, like toothpaste, antibacterial soap, deodorant, and hand wash are reported to have this chemical.

Realizing the growing evidence of endocrine disruptive properties and the environmental impact including contribution to antimicrobial resistance, many big companies have voluntarily started measures for phasing out use these chemicals. The products with label "Do not contain triclosan" are available. Now it is the turn of companies in India to take steps not to use them in public interest. The Indian Drugs Control Authority must issue the users' advice in the light of USFDA's ruling. USFDA allowed the companies a year time to comply with its ruling of not permitting the use of the chemicals in soaps and washes. The use of these antibacterial agents would continue in hand sanitizers and antibacterial products for healthcare setting.

In absence of immediate actions from the regulatory authorities or voluntary users' guidance from the companies, one must avoid the use of antibacterial soaps and washes in one's own and public interest. Washing with plain soap and running water remains one of the most important steps to avoid getting sick and to prevent spreading germs to others. Washing hands physically removes germs by friction. While regular washing with soap and running water is adequate for individual at home, hand washing with antibacterial agents may be essential in hospitals.

(m) Body Mass Index (BMI) – Your Health Barometer!

All of us are fascinated by the attractive images of young women and men projected in media as models. Conscious general populations start comparing their weight and often get dissatisfied being unable to resemble these ideal figures. Many are unhappy about their weight (Overweight and often Obesity). This overweight not only just declines individual's self esteem but also a cause of concern of his/her health.

The obesity is a strong predictor of high prevalence of diabetes, hypertension and coronary artery diseases. It has been reported that India would be the world's diabetes capital by 2050. The current statistics shows the prevalence of diabetes mellitus is around 118 per thousand for urban and 38 per thousand for rural population. The prevalence of hypertension is also reported to be around 160 per thousand. Obesity is also known to have associated with other diseases like gastro esophageal disease. Even it influences the medicines' action through regulating their distribution within the body.

About 30-50 percent adult Indians are either overweight or obese. The imbalance between the energy intake and energy output leads to excess accumulation of in various parts of the body leading to overweight and obesity. There are several techniques like weight to hip ratio, height – weight tables, body mass index (BMI), and electrical impedance available to determine ideal or healthy body weight for the individuals. The body mass index is the most popular among the techniques and has been used by World Health Organization as standards for recording obesity almost for last thirty years.

The Body Mass Index (BMI) indicates the relationship of body weight (expressed in kilogram) to height (expressed in meter) of the individuals. This can be obtained by dividing body weight by the square of height and expressed in kilogram per square meter.

$$\text{BMI} = \frac{\text{weight (kg)}}{\text{height}^2\ \left(\text{m}^2\right)}$$

BMI can also be obtained from charts of weight and height. Realizing the issues of obesity, the Government of India revised the weight and flab statistics. Indians are different from their western counterparts both in body composition and genetics. People in India suffer from abdominal obesity; in contrast the people of west are uniformly obese. The distribution of fat around the abdomen is considered to be more harmful than fat around the hips. The body composition of Indians put them in high risk of diabetes and high blood pressure. The indicatives of BMI are:

BMI is equal to or less than 18.5 (Under Weight): This indicates under weight. They need to consult physician to explore gaining weight as low body mass decreases immune system leading to illness.

BMI is between 18.5 and 23 (Normal): This reflects the ideal body weight. They are likely to have lower incidence of serious illness than people with higher or lower BMI. They look physically more attractive. [WHO guideline requires 18.5 to 25 as ideal weight].

BMI is between 25 and 29.9 (Over Weight): The value reflects over weight. Individuals who fall in this range are at increased risk for a variety of illness. They need to follow healthy ways to lower their weight, such as diet and exercise.

BMI is over 30 (Obese): This indicates a physically unhealthy condition which puts the persons at risk for serious illnesses such as heart disease, diabetes, high blood pressure, gall bladder disease, and some cancers. These persons would benefit greatly by modifying their lifestyle.

The categorization of BMI for obesity is different for children and adolescents. The BMI provides a simple numeric measure of a person's fatness or thinness that allows health professionals to discuss the overweight or underweight problems of patients more objectively. BMI is a good indicator of risk of morbidity and mortality in young and middle aged adults. BMI can predict the underlying risks in a large population and can be used as an early warning sign that can suggest if lifestyle changes are required or not. About 33 percent of adult men and 36 percent of women have BMI below 18.5 indicating chronic energy deficiency. The body image problem of extremely thin people is also equally distressing. They too require appropriate nutrition like overweight and obese persons.

(n) Disposing Unused or Expired Medicines

It is necessary to properly dispose of your expired, unwanted or unused medicines. If not disposed properly, it may harm others or even cause environmental issues. In case of difficulties, you should consult your pharmacist who has the expertise on medicines. If possible, it is to be returned to the seller or donate to charity.

The medicines at household level are disposed in two ways:

(i) **Flushing medicines:** The unused or expired medicines are to be flushed them down the sink or toilet.

(ii) **Disposing medicines in household trash:** Almost all medicines can be thrown into your household trash. These include prescription and over-the-counter (OTC) drugs in pills, liquids, drops, patches, creams, and inhalers.

Here are the general guidelines (Source USFDA):

1. Remove the drugs from their original containers and mix them with something undesirable, such as used coffee grounds, dirt, or cat litter. This makes the medicine less appealing to children and pets and unrecognizable to someone who might intentionally go through the trash looking for drugs.
2. Put the mixture in something you can close (a re-sealable zipper storage bag, empty can, or other container) to prevent the drug from leaking or spilling out.
3. Throw the container in the garbage.
4. Scratch out all your personal information on the empty medicine packaging to protect your identity and privacy. Throw the packaging away.

Some prescription drugs — such as powerful narcotic pain medicines and other controlled substances — have instructions for flushing to reduce the danger of overdose from unintentional or illegal use.

Disposing of Inhaler Products

One environmental concern involves inhalers used by people who have asthma or other breathing problems, such as chronic obstructive pulmonary disease. Read handling instructions on the labelling of inhalers and aerosol products. These products could be dangerous if punctured or thrown into a fire or incinerator.

(o) Wash Your Hands of Hazards

Millions of people die each year due to various hospital related issues. The hospital related issues are mainly attributed to the medical errors and hospital acquired infections. Of every 100 hospitalized patients 7 in developed countries and 10 in developing countries usually acquire hospital acquired infection. Longer the patients stay in hospital, higher is the risk with the patients of getting infected. Many times these infections are of multi drug resistant organisms and are not only difficult to treat but the treatment often expensively prohibited.

In a recent report on antimicrobial resistance (AMR) the World Health Organization (WHO) cautions that the AMR is no longer a prediction of the future. It has been occurring right now in every region of the world and has the potential to affect every one, of any age, in any country. WHO calls for combined strategies to combat antimicrobial resistance. Hand washing is advocated as one of the prime strategies. Hand washing with soap and water is among the most effective and inexpensive ways to prevent diarrhoeal diseases and pneumonia. Diarrhoea and Pneumonia are the major killer diseases for deaths under five. As hands are the principal carriers of disease causing germs, it is necessary that everyone should wash hands with soap and water before feeding children, after toileting, before taking food etc.

In USA 1.7 million infections are acquired in hospital causing 100,000 deaths every year. In Europe, there are about 4.5 million infections causing 37,000 deaths every year. However, as we do not have a surveillance and documenting system, there are no data for our country. While the hand washing by the individuals promotes health and reduces the chances of infection, the good hand washing practices by the health workers help reducing the transmission of hospital acquired infection. Simple hand washing with water does not serve the real purpose. The principal of cleaning is to remove visible dirt. Dirt and grease carry most germs. It is essentially a mechanical process but the use of soap helps removing the dirt quickly due to its solubilizing effect. Cleaning has to be carried out in a standardized manner to ensure an adequate level of cleanliness. The World Health Organization every year campaigns for Save Lives: Clean Your Hands. This year it focuses on combating AMR through good hand hygiene practices.

Studies have shown that good hand hygiene practices adopted by the health care professionals cause substantial decrease of multi drug resistant organism's infection. In resource constraint situations the hand hygiene gets low priority at least in general wards of the hospitals. The government must ensure sensitizing the health care workers and providing adequate facilities for hand washing after examination or handling of each patient to prevent hospital acquired infection not only in patient's safety but also from economic point. The total costs of hand hygiene promotion correspond to less than 1% of the costs associated with hospital acquired infection.

"Going into hospital is far riskier than flying." Someone once says. The risk of dying in air crash is estimated to be around 1 in 10 million passengers while the chances of dying from hospital related issues could be 1 in 300. "Do the doctors clean their hands prior to examining patients" may be an indicator for checking quality service when next time you think of a hospital!

(p) Pop Up But Know Them Well!

The two recent incidents of medicine mishap have created lot of concerns among the people. After taking iron tablets in schools, several children of two districts of Odisha were reported to have fallen sick and were admitted to hospitals. Several children were admitted to hospital after a vaccine mix up in Bengal. The two cases are different but both have harmed the children. In the first case, children were ignorant of the medicines they are given and they had taken more than one tablet at a time that too in empty stomach (perhaps they had taken food much before) in the schools. In the latter case, children were given hepatitis B vaccine drops in place of polio drops. It is difficult to understand how drops can be obtained from hepatitis B vials.

Iron tablets (often along with folic acid) are distributed among young children under national Nutritional Anaemia prophylaxis programme. The programme is now part of Reproductive and Child Health (RCH) programme. Anaemia is a severe public health issue in the country. The iron deficiency anaemia reduces the work capacity of individuals and populations leading to serious economic consequences and become the obstacle for nation development. Although anaemia level may vary, anaemia is wide spread among children in almost all states and iron supplementation is one of the several strategies adopted to address this anaemia issue. Iron has the metallic taste and is not palatable. Ferrous sulphate is the preferred iron salt as it easily absorbs. But it undergoes oxidation in presence of air forming ferric salts. The ferric salts are not absorbable. In order to overcome the two issues: taste and stability, the tablets are sugar coated. The sugar coated tablets are often mistaken as candies and overdosing toxicity is often common in children. They are required to be kept out of reach of children. Unfortunately, we do have no such awareness nor we have child resistant containers. The iron is known to cause gastric irritation and to avoid or prevent this; they are required to be taken after meals. But no one has cautioned the children!

The medicines are important to all of us. But they are like double edged weapons. They may harm us if not used properly. It has been estimated that adverse drug events are responsible for 5% hospitalization in high income and 2.9% in low and middle income countries. The World Health Organization estimated that more than 50% of the people do not take the medicines appropriately. One of the main reasons of not taking medicines correctly is lack of understanding of the recommended medicines. It is necessary to know the medicines that are given or prescribed for us. More we know, better do they work. Make sure to know your medicines before you use them. Your doctor and pharmacist do help you knowing more about your medicines. Though internet has been widely used to have access to information, but one needs to select the reliable sources. There are many misleading sites.

You must know at least the following before you start taking or using medicines:

- Name of the medicine and its purpose.
- Dose – how many and at what time.
- When to take – after food or before food? / How to use?
- What to do if a dose is missed?
- How long to be taken and when to stop?
- What are the side effects – if you experience what to do?
- Whether certain foods or drinks are to be avoided?
- Whether other medicines currently taking are to be avoided?
- How to store at home?

Unsafe medicine use, where the patients are harmed by the medicines designed to help them, can have wide range of consequences. People may lose the trust on the health workers or health facilities. Even the quality of medicines is questioned.

INDEX

C

D

E

F

G

H

I

K

L

M

N

O

P

U

V

W

X

Z

www.ingramcontent.com/pod-product-compliance
Ingram Content Group UK Ltd.
Pitfield, Milton Keynes, MK11 3LW, UK
UKHW021328190726
13845UKWH00004B/81

9 789388 305655